POCKET SE[RIES]
MRCP PART 2

BOOK 3

Haematology, Rheumatology
and
Neurology

POCKET SERIES FOR MRCP PART 2

BOOK 3
Haematology, Rheumatology and Neurology

Edited by Richard L. Hawkins MBBS FRCS

Haematology:
Anne Yardumian MD MRCP MRCPath
The North Middlesex Hospital, London

Helen C. Kelsey BSc MB BS MRCP
The Middlesex Hospital

Rheumatology:
Elaine Baguley MB BS MRCP
St Thomas' Hospital, London

Neurology:
Christopher M. C. Allen, MA MD MRCP
Addenbrooke's Hospital, Cambridge

© 1990 PASTEST
Egerton Court, Parkgate Estate, Knutsford
Cheshire WA16 0ED
Tel: 01565 755226

All rights reserved. No part of this publication may be reproduced, stored in a retrieval system, or transmitted, in any form or by any means, electronic, mechanical, photocopying, recording or otherwise without the prior permission of the copyright owner.

First printed in 1990
Reprinted 1995

A catalogue reference for this title is available from the British Library.

ISBN 0 906896 47 9

Text prepared by Turner Associates, Knutsford, Cheshire
Phototypeset by Speedset Ltd, Ellesmere Port, Cheshire
Printed in Great Britain by BPC Wheatons Ltd, Exeter.

CONTENTS

INTRODUCTION vii

HAEMATOLOGY
  Case Histories (6) 1
  Data Interpretations (12) 13

RHEUMATOLOGY
  Case Histories (6) 29
  Data Interpretations (14) 35

NEUROLOGY
  Case Histories (7) 59
  Data Interpretations (14) 73

Answers and teaching notes are on the reverse of each question page.

INDEX 87

INTRODUCTION

The MRCP Part 2 Examination is a test of competent clinical practice as opposed to the theoretical knowledge required for Part 1. The examiners want to be reassured that the candidate is professional in his or her approach and manner, accomplished in technique, safe in practice and honest in ignorance. There is no doubt that efficient, systematic preparation for the Part 2 can make all the difference between passing and failing the examination. Familiarity with the type of questions being set, together with a knowledge of how best to present the answers and how they are marked by the examiners, will all help candidates to do their best in the examination.

Each of these three PasTest pocket books contain sample case histories and data interpretations carefully written and edited by doctors involved in the teaching and preparation of candidates for the MRCP examination. The case material, data and questions presented have all been chosen for their similarity to those experienced in recent official examinations:

Book 1: Cardiology and Respiratory Medicine
Book 2: Gastroenterology, Endocrinology and Renal Medicine
Book 3: Haematology, Rheumatology and Neurology.

The best way to use these books is to work through each question in a methodical manner keeping to the time limits set by the Royal College. This will give useful practice in coming to quick decisions about the answers, which can then be looked up, corrected and thought about in a more leisurely manner.

By working through these books and studying the correct answers and teaching notes, a candidate will be able to pinpoint specific topics and subject areas where further reading and study would be beneficial before the examination. **Please note that the correct answers given in these books are not presented in a simple list as required by the College on examination day, but are incorporated within the teaching notes.**

The written section of the examination consists of three question papers:

(a) Case Histories (four or more compulsory questions in 55 minutes.)
(b) Data Interpretation (ten compulsory questions in 45 minutes.)
(c) Projected Material (twenty compulsory questions in 40 minutes.)

The Royal College has published a booklet of 2 past MRCP Part 2 written examinations (general medicine and paediatrics) and all candidates would be wise to be familiar with these, in particular the simple answer format preferred.

Introduction

Advice on How to Answer the Questions

The written part of the MRCP Part 2 examination has been designed to require minimal writing so that maximum time may be devoted by the candidate to thinking through the problems presented while, at the same time, it allows for objective marking by the examiners. This means that marks are awarded by the examiners in a predetermined manner. Specific answers are required and so candidates must listen carefully to the invigilator's instructions and understand exactly how to present their answers. Since specific answers are required, it is of no use to treat the questions as short answer questions in which you attempt to explain your thoughts to the examiner. Answers should be precise, yet complete, in their meaning. Vague answers score significantly lower marks.

Each question asks for a specific number of answers. Correct answers to a question will receive maximum marks but since there may be more than one possible correct answer, marks will be awarded on a scale according to their acceptability. Where the 'best' answer is much better than the others, the difference in marking between the best and the other answers will be greater. Answers in excess of the number requested will be ignored. For example, if three diagnoses are given instead of two, only the first two will be marked, even if the third represents the best response. Space is given in the examination paper for each of your answers and it will be of considerable help to the examiners if you confine your answers to one per line.

All three papers in the written section are ascribed the same maximum number of marks. The final score for each candidate is the aggregate mark of all three papers. In order to pass, it is not necessary therefore to obtain a pass mark in each of the three papers, so long as the aggregate mark reaches the required pass mark.

Candidates who pass the written section are invited to attend for further examination in the clinical and oral sections. Those who marginally fail the written section may also proceed to the clinical and oral sections but, to succeed in the examination as a whole, have to obtain additional marks in these last two sections.

Candidates who have clearly failed the written section are deemed to have failed the examination as a whole and must resit the written section in order to proceed in the examination.

It is hoped that the material provided in these three pocket books will prove instrumental in the success of many Part 2 candidates.

HAEMATOLOGY : CASE HISTORIES

1. A 48 year old Punjabi businessman reported to his GP that he had noticed a painless swelling on the left side of his neck over the preceding 6 weeks. There had also been some similar but tender lumps on the other side of his neck. On direct questioning he had also noticed some weight loss of one stone in eight months though he had previously been, and still was overweight. He also had a non-productive cough, minor shortness of breath, and some night-time sweats. He smoked 30 cigarettes daily and drank no alcohol. He frequently travelled to all parts of the world on business, and three weeks previously had been in the Punjab. There was no relevant family or past medical history, and apart from an isolated 2 x 2 cm firm node in the left supraclavicular fossa there were no abnormal clinical findings.

His presenting results were:

Hb	11.2 g/dl
RBC	4.5 x 10^{12}/l
MCV	77 fl
WBC	14.5 X 10^9/l, 58% neutrophils, 33% lymphocytes, 9% eosinophils
ESR	47 mm in first hour

Urea and electrolytes, liver function tests, calcium and albumin – all within normal ranges.

Questions:

1. What diagnoses would you consider possible? Give five.

2. What investigations would you request?

Answers overleaf

Case Histories : Answers

1. 1. Infective causes, which would account for the previous more widespread lymphadenopathy, should be considered for example, viral, or more rare atypical organisms such as toxoplasma. Tuberculosis is a real possibility and must be sought. The symptoms and enlarged node might be the presentation for a non-haematological malignancy such as bronchogenic or gastric neoplasm. Hodgkin's disease or non-Hodgkin's lymphoma must be considered; the latter is less likely to present as isolated lymphadenopathy, but can do so, especially the higher grade types. One should not be put off the possibility of malignant lymphadenopathy by the history of preceding more widespread node enlargement: people frequently only notice one enlarged node when other tender nodes are present caused, for example, by incidental viral infection. Sarcoidosis could also present in this way.

2. Investigations required include: viral antibody screen, toxoplasma serology, sputum plus urine examination for evidence of tuberculosis, chest X-ray. A Mantoux test might be informative: a positive result would be expected in this man and so such a result would be inconclusive; if negative one might suspect impaired cell-mediated immunity. The most important investigation, however, given the systemic symptoms which accompany the enlarged node in this man, is excision biopsy of the involved node.

2. Mr E. C., a 68 year old Caucasian man, presented to his GP with an episode of gastroenteritis nine months ago. At the time, examination revealed a spleen tip palpable 4 cm below the costal margin. He gave a history of at least two attacks of malaria while in north Africa during the war. He was otherwise well and the symptoms resolved rapidly without specific treatment. No investigations were performed, the splenomegaly being attributed to previous recurrent malaria. He now presents having noted increasing tiredness over the last 3 weeks, and a cough with pleuritic chest pains and fevers for five days. He smokes 20 cigarettes and drinks three pints of beer daily. Examination shows a very unwell man, fever 38.2°C, with a herpetic lesion on the lower lip. He has signs of consolidation in the left lower zone of the chest, and enlarged liver (three cm) and spleen (8 cm).

His blood count shows the following:

Hb	8.8 g/dl
WBC	53.7 x 10^9/l, 39% neutrophils, 9% metamyelocytes, 22% myelocytes, 3% promyelocytes, 24% blast cells, 3% nucleated red cells
Platelets	33 x 10^9/l.

Questions:

1. What diagnoses would you consider to explain the haematological findings? Give five.

2. Give five relevant haematological investigations to differentiate between the diagnoses.

Answers overleaf

Case Histories : Answers

2. 1. The man has evidence of pneumonia, and a high white count with marked 'left shift' (primitive cells in the peripheral blood). The combination of erythroid precursors (the nucleated red cells) and myeloid left shift is termed a leuco-erythroblastic blood film. He might have a primary haematological illness with impaired immunity giving rise to his current infection. This could be acute leukaemia (myeloblastic or lymphoblastic) arising de novo although the preserved, indeed increased, mature neutrophil count does not support this diagnosis. Chronic myeloid leukaemia presenting in transformation (too high a blast count for chronic phase) would account for all the haematological findings and the relatively longstanding splenomegaly, as would myelofibrosis, although the percentage of blasts is rather higher than usually seen; characteristic red cell changes like tear drop poikilocytes should be sought on the blood film. Alternatively, he may have a non-haematological malignancy with bone marrow involvement; in view of his pneumonia and smoking history a bronchogenic tumour is possible. Again the blast count is rather high, but a degree of leuco-erythroblastic change on the blood film is classically seen in marrow infiltration by such disease. Finally the elevated WBC with left shift and occasional nucleated red cells might be attributable to a stressed marrow response to his pneumonia, thus a reactive not a malignant problem, a so-called 'leukaemoid reaction'.

2. Investigations to differentiate between these diagnoses should include bone marrow aspirate and trephine biopsy. The acute leukaemias would be evidenced by a marrow blast count of >30%, myelofibrosis gives a difficult or dry tap with increased reticulin on the trephine. Other malignant cells, if present, should be identifiable in clumps on the marrow aspirate. Conventional cytochemistry and immunophenotyping of the blasts in the blood or marrow will differentiate between myeloid and lymphoid blasts. Chromosome analysis frequently provides clues in the diagnosis of haematological malignancy. Whether the neutrophilia with left shift is part of a reactive or malignant process can frequently be clarified with a leucocyte alkaline phosphatase stain. If reactive, the neutrophils stain strongly giving a high score (they may do so in myelofibrosis also), whereas in chronic granulocytic leukaemia and sometimes in acute myeloblastic leukaemia the score is very low.

Haematology : Case Histories

3. Mrs C. L., a 33 year old Caucasian woman, first presented with a pneumonic illness and pleurisy two years ago. She was previously on no medication and is a non-smoker. While in hospital she developed an extensive ileo-femoral thrombosis and was treated with six months of warfarin anticoagulation.

Pre-treatment investigations showed:

Hb	11.8 g/dl
WBC	23.6 x 10^9/l, 81% neutrophils with a mild left shift
Platelets	131 x 10^9/l
PT	15 (control 13 seconds)
APTT	79 (control 34 seconds;
Thrombin time	12 (control 13 seconds)

APTT 50:50 mix with normal plasma : 66 seconds

Questions:

1. What diagnosis do you suspect to account for her clinical presentation and clotting derangement?

2. What investigations would you carry out to confirm your suspicion?

One year later, after waking one morning she noticed a 'dark blob' in front of her right eye. She went to a local eye hospital, where an isolated haemorrhage was noted adjacent to a branch of the upper temporal branch of the right retinal vein. No other retinopathy was evident. This was slow to resolve, and at a further attendance her blood pressure was checked and found to be 150/100. This was confirmed on two subsequent occasions, with diastolic pressures between 95 and 100 mm Hg.

Question:

3. What management would you now advise for her eye complication?

Answers overleaf

Case Histories : Answers

3. 1. The woman had a high WBC count and neutrophilia, in keeping with her acute pulmonary illness. She has also demonstrated a thrombotic tendency. In the light of subsequent events her initial chest presentation may have represented a pulmonary embolus with secondary infection, or could have been a primary infection with thrombotic problems secondary to immobilisation. Such a presentation in a young woman should raise the possibility of a 'connective tissue disorder', of which there is more evidence in this patient. She has a prolonged APTT, which fails to correct when the test is repeated on a 1:1 mixture of her plasma with pooled normal plasma: this points to an inhibitor of coagulation, as opposed to a factor deficiency as the cause of the long APTT. These findings plus the thrombotic tendency are strongly suggestive of a 'lupus-type anticoagulant'. This is directed against phospholipid, and gives rise clinically to a hyper-coagulable state while producing paradoxically prolonged clotting times (especially APTT) in vitro.

2. An autoantibody screen/anti DNA antibodies will help to elucidate whether she has systemic lupus erythematosus. Renal functions tests will also be necessary. Coagulation tests to confirm the presence of a lupus-type inhibitor should be carried out: several are available. The 'dilute thromboplastin test' is one of the simpler ones; PT's are repeated on the patient's plasma using a series of dilutions of the thromboplastin. This is the source of phospholipid in this test, so in the presence of this inhibitor the concentration of reagent becomes critical as it is diluted, and the PT prolongs excessively at each dilution compared to the same dilutions of thromboplastin in the presence of control plasma. The 'dilute Russell's Viper venom test' is a more specific test. Assays for anti-cardiolipin antibodies should also be carried out.

3. The degree of hypertension documented is modest, and in the absence of any other retinopathy, is unlikely to be the cause of this lady's retinal haemorrhage. In view of her history, and diagnosis of SLE plus lupus anti-coagulant it is more likely that she had a branch retinal vein thrombosis with secondary vessel leakage. She should be started on an anti-thrombotic agent: low dose aspirin (300 mg twice a week or 75 mg daily) is probably as effective as any in this condition.

Haematology : Case Histories

4. A 48 year old man presented to his GP complaining of decreased libido and erectile impotence. He was an insulin dependent diabetic of four years standing and had a history of heavy alcohol intake although he had apparently reduced this somewhat recently. He was on no medication apart from insulin. On examination he looked plethoric and there was a smell of alcohol on his breath. There was no finger clubbing or jaundice. Spider naevi were present over his chest and axillary and pubic hair were reduced. His chest was clear. Abdominal examination revealed 6 cm hepatomegaly, but no ascites. Examination of the fundi, cranial nerves and peripheral nervous system were normal.

Investigations showed:

Hb		15.2 g/dl
WBC		7.9×10^9/l
RBC		5.1×10^{12}/l
MCV		102 fl
MCH		28 pg
MCHC		28 g/dl
PCV		52%
Plasma	sodium	136 mmol/l
	potassium	4.0 mmol/l
	urea	6.2 mmol/l
	bilirubin	32 µmol/l
Serum	IgG	24 g/l
	IgA	2.5 g/l
	IgM	1.2 g/l
	albumin	35 g/l
	total protein	80 g/l
	glutamyl transferase	200 iu/l
Blood	glucose	11.8 mmol/l
Random blood alcohol level		10 mmol/l
Autoantibody screen and ANF		negative

Questions:

1. Suggest two causes for the deranged liver function.

2. Suggest five further investigations to aid the differential diagnosis.

Answers overleaf

Case Histories : Answers

4. 1. The combination of liver damage, insulin dependency and gonadal dysfunction suggest parenchymal tissue damage secondary to iron overload, and in this context primary or idiopathic haemochromatosis (IH) must be considered. Alcohol abuse with ensuing liver disease could give rise to many of the features seen but the insulin dependency is very suggestive of iron overload.

2. In alcoholic liver disease serum iron and transferrin saturation may be greatly increased as in IH, although almost total transferrin saturation is suggestive of the latter. Serum ferritin is raised in both. Liver biopsy may help to differentiate the conditions. In IH there is evidence of greatly increased iron (which can be quantified) which is chiefly parenchymal (i.e. inside the hepatocytes themselves). In alcoholic liver disease, as well as other suggestive features on liver biopsy, the iron tends to be confined to the Kuppfer cells and loading is usually less extreme. The desferrioxamine (DFO) excretion test, whereby the iron content of urine excreted over 24 hours after an injection of 500 mg of DFO is quantified, can give a useful guide to the total body iron content.

Haematology : Case Histories

5. A 65 year old Caucasian presented with an episode of haematemesis and melaena stools. There was no preceding history of indigestion or gastro-intestinal haemorrhage. Three years previously he had undergone trans-urethral prostatectomy, recovery from which had been complicated by a deep venous thrombosis in the right leg for which he had received warfarin for three months. He was on no medication, smoked five cigarettes per day and drank one or two pints of beer daily. On examination, he looked pale, not jaundiced, and there was no lymphadenopathy. Blood pressure 120/75 mm Hg, pulse 92/min regular, JVP not elevated, chest clear. Abdominal examination revealed a palpable spleen tip with no other abnormal findings.
Investigations showed:

Hb	11.8 g/dl
WBC	18.6 x 10^9/l, 92% neutrophils
	7% lymphocytes
	1% monocytes
RBC	5.6 x 10^{12}/l
MCV	67 fl
MCH	21 pg
MCHC	29 g/dl
Platelets	854 x 10^9/l
Plasma sodium	138 mmol/l
potassium	4.5 mmol/l
urea	16.6 mmol/l
Serum creatinine	118 μmol/l
calcium	2.32 mmol/l
phosphate	1.21 mmol/l
albumin	36 g/l
urate	460 μmol/l
aspartate transaminase	54 iu/l
alkaline phosphatase	210 iu/ml
glutamyl transferase	200 iu/l

The bleeding settled spontaneously. Upper gastro-intestinal endoscopy showed a small pre-pyloric ulcer with evidence of recent bleeding, biopsy confirmed a benign gastric ulcer.

Questions:
1. What diagnoses would you consider to explain this man's haematological abnormalities?
2. Why is the urea raised with a relatively normal creatinine?
3. What further four investigations would you perform?

Answers overleaf

Case Histories : Answers

5. 1. The haematological abnormalities are: mild microcytic anaemia, a considerably raised platelet count and a neutrophilia. These abnormalities could all be reactive, secondary to chronic subclinical blood loss from his peptic ulcer and resulting iron deficiency, with an acute bleed superimposed. However, there are clues that it may not be this simple: these are the palpable spleen and the fact that despite a significantly low MCV, the haemoglobin reduction is only mild and the RBC count is normal. These features raise the possibility of a myeloproliferative disorder, in which case the platelet count and neutrophilia may be primary and were it not for concomitant iron deficiency, his haemoglobin would probably be raised also (i.e. there is an element of polycythaemia being 'held down' by iron deficiency). Iron deficiency is frequently seen in the myeloproliferative disorders, because occult gastro-intestinal blood loss is common and also because frank peptic ulceration is a recognised complication of these disorders. As frequently, there is evidence in this man of involvement of all three cell lines in the myeloproliferative process, but the thrombocyctosis is the most marked and so he would probably be labelled 'essential thrombocythaemia' (ET).
2. The raised urea with almost normal creatinine is the result of his upper gastro-intestinal haemorrhage with resulting large 'protein load' in the gut. These findings are characteristic and may be useful diagnostically for example in detecting re-bleeding.
3. Examination of a blood film may confirm iron deficient features; and platelet anisocytosis with large abnormally staining forms would be in favour of myeloproliferative disorder rather than reactive thrombocytosis. His iron status should also be confirmed biochemically (serum Fe/TIBC or ferritin). Bone marrow examination may be useful: it would be hypercellular in either condition, in ET additionally atypical megakaryocyte forms may be seen and there is often increased reticulin on the trephine biopsy. Chromosome studies on marrow cells would be most useful as abnormalities of karyotype are frequently seen in ET and related disorders and sometimes a Philadelphia chromosome is found raising the possibility of an atypical presentation of chronic granulocytic leukaemia. Formal platelet aggregation studies are useful in thrombocytosis: the abnormalities in ET and other myeloproliferative disorders are complex, and this is reflected by the fact that bleeding or thrombotic complications can be seen in the same individual at different times, as in this man. Spontaneous aggregation may be seen, i.e. a marker of increased platelet activity, but in vitro responses to adrenaline and collagen as stimulating agents are commonly subnormal.

Haematology : Case Histories

5. A 74 year old widower complained of progressive shortness of breath associated with increasing fatigue. He recently had a course of antibiotics from his GP for a chest infection. He complained of occasional indigestion but had noted no blood in his stool or melaena. There was no history of haematuria, haemoptyses or other apparent source of blood loss. His general health was good with steady weight and good appetite. He was an ex-smoker and drank very little alcohol. Regular medication consisted of a diuretic for hypertension. His only other complaint was of longstanding backache.

On examination he was pale, no lymphadenopathy, BP 140/80 mm Hg, chest clear, abdominal examination unremarkable.

Investigations showed:

Hb	8.5 g/dl
WBC	9.5×10^9/l
RBC	5.1×10^{12}/l
MCV	71 fl
MCH	16.5 pg
MCHC	23.1 g/dl
PCV	37.7%
Platelets	485×10^9/l
Plasma sodium	138 mmol/l
potassium	4.1 mmol/l
urea	7.2 mmol/l
Serum creatinine	120 µmol/l
albumin	37 g/l
total protein	95 g/l

INR 1.23

Film: microcytic hypochromic, some rouleaux noted
Serum electrophoresis: M-band in the γ-region

Questions:

1. What four investigations are needed to characterise the anaemia further?

2. What five investigations are needed to characterise the M-band further?

Answers overleaf

Case Histories : Answers

6. 1. The picture is one of microcytic hypochromic anaemia. Iron deficiency is the likeliest cause and the blood film should be studied and serum iron and total iron binding capacity should be measured. A dietary history and search for a site of chronic occult blood loss should be sought, especially in the gastrointestinal tract. Faecal occult blood tests may confirm blood loss and then upper and lower GI investigations (barium studies and/or endoscopy) must be pursued. Rectal examination and sigmoidoscopy are imperative.

2. The other finding in this man is of a monoclonal band on serum protein electrophoresis. While this may be contributing to his anaemia (for example on the basis of myeloma) this diagnosis cannot be made on the basis of the M-band alone as about 3% of individuals over 70 years of age have one. The problem is to distinguish between 'monoclonal gammopathy of uncertain significance' (MGUS) and myeloma or other malignant disease with paraprotein (e.g. Waldenstrom's macroglobulinaemia or chronic lymphatic leukaemia). Evaluation of the M-band should include: inspection of a blood film, characterisation of the paraprotein by immunoelectrophoresis (viz IgG/M/A and κ or λ), its quantitation, quantitation of other immunoglobulin subclasses, renal function tests, plasma calcium and phosphate, β2-microglobulin assay, urine study to look for Bence Jones proteinuria, skeletal survey, bone marrow aspiration and trephine biopsy.

HAEMATOLOGY : DATA INTERPRETATIONS

1. A 22 year old Caucasian female patient is referred by her GP with a week's history of a sore mouth, malaise, and fevers to 38.5°C. She has previously been entirely well except for occasional headaches, for which she takes some proprietary analgesia.

   Her blood count is:

Hb	8.8 g/dl
MCV	75 fl
WBC	$0.8 \times 10^9/l$, 94% lymphocytes, no blasts seen
Platelets	$18 \times 10^9/l$

   Reticulocyte count 0.1% (absolute reticulocyte count $14 \times 10^9/l$)

   Questions:

   1. What diagnoses would you consider? Give three possibilities.

   2. What investigations would you immediately organise? List four.

   3. What treatment would you commence immediately?

   4. What is the significance of the reticulocyte count?

Answers overleaf

Data Interpretations : Answers

1. 1. This girl is pancytopenic, with severe neutropenia (<6% of 0.8 x 10^9/l) and marked thrombocytopenia, with evidence of infection (significant pyrexia).
   The likeliest diagnoses are acute leukaemia, despite the absence of blasts in the peripheral blood, or bone marrow aplasia which might be idiopathic, or secondary to drug therapy, for example certain analgesics related to amidopyrine are particularly noted for this. Viral induced bone marrow suppression can occur as a temporary phenomenon for example with Epstein Barr virus infection, but the counts are rarely so severely depressed. Consumption cytopenias, for example on an auto-immune basis, are less likely and the low reticulocyte count would be against this.

   2. The diagnosis must be urgently clarified and in particular the source of infection sought in this severely neutropenic girl. Blood cultures, viral swabs of the mouth/throat and an MSU must be organised immediately, viral antibody titres and chest X-ray might be helpful in addition. A bone marrow aspirate and trephine biopsy are mandatory to make a diagnosis so that appropriate treatment can be commenced. A 'monospot' test should be checked.

   3. Treatment must be started with intravenous broad spectrum antibiotics immediately, without waiting for the results of any of the above tests, as infection can be rapidly fatal in the absence of neutrophils. Gentamicin plus piperacillin, or ceftazidime, are suitable until culture results are available, when appropriate alterations to cover any specific organisms can be made. Anti-viral therapy with acyclovir would be indicated if there is evidence of herpes infection in the painful mouth. If there is evidence of infection with candida oral anti-fungals should be started and some should be commenced anyway on a pro-phylactic basis. If leukaemia is diagnosed, allopurinol should be started immediately in preparation for commencing chemotherapy, in anticipation of rapid cell kill.

   4. The reticulocyte percentage is low in the face of anaemia, and the absolute reticulocyte count is reduced (normal range 20–100 x 10^9/l). This indicates production failure rather than excessive consumption as a cause of the anaemia. If the diagnosis proves to be aplastic anaemia, this low reticulocyte count, together with the presenting neutrophil count of below 0.5 x 10^9/l and platelets below 20 x 10^9/l, puts this girl into a poor prognostic group.

2. A 5 year old Caucasian boy is brought to his GP because he has been lethargic and uninterested in anything for three or four days, and his mother thinks he looks pale. She also reports that he and his brother both had a mild febrile illness seven to ten days previously from which he had recovered before the lethargy started, and his brother was now entirely well again. On examination, the child is sleepy and very pale, there is a palpable spleen tip.

His blood count shows:

Hb	4.2 g/dl
MCV	80 fl
MCH	31 pg
MCHC	38 g/dl
Reticulocytes	0.3%
WBC	6.4 x 10^9/l, 69% lymphocytes of unremarkable morphology
Platelets	263 x 10^9/l

Questions:

1. What is the most likely precipitating cause for such a presentation?

2. What might be the underlying haematological diagnosis in this boy and what investigations would you do to confirm this?

Answers overleaf

Data Interpretations : Answers

2. 1. The striking abnormality is the profound anaemia and accompanying very low reticulocyte count. This indicates failure of erythropoiesis as the cause for the anaemia. The WBC and platelet counts are well preserved (the relative lymphocytosis is normal for his age), so the problem is confined to the erythroid series. The viral illness seven to ten days previously has provoked the problem: many viruses can cause a mild transient bone marrow depression, but profound red cell aplasia is frequently attributable to parvovirus, or B19 virus.

2. In all individuals with such an infection there is transient arrest of erythroid activity, normally this leads to a minor, if detectable, fall in haemoglobin before the marrow recovers. However, people whose red cell survival is already much reduced cannot tolerate such a 'switch-off' in erythropoiesis, as they depend on increased erythroid activity to maintain their steady state haemoglobin. Such individuals include those with some of the haemoglobinopathies (e.g. sickle cell disease), enzymopathies (e.g. pyruvate kinase deficiency) and those with red cell membrane defects (e.g. hereditary spherocytosis). Adult patients with acquired haemolytic anaemias can suffer similarly. The child described probably has hereditary spherocytosis (HS), the clue being the raised MCHC, characteristic of spherocytic cells which have a degree of intracellular dehydration due to ion leakage through the abnormal membrane.

The diagnosis of HS can be confirmed by inspection of a blood film and by osmotic fragility tests. Spherocytes, having a lower surface area:volume ratio, can accommodate less additional water than normal cells and so lyse in less hypotonic saline solution. Family studies may also be useful: the disease is transmitted as an autosomal dominant.

Haematology : Data Interpretations

3. A 36 year old Asian male patient presents with tiredness, some headaches and the following blood count:

Hb	9.2 g/dl
MCV	109 fl
WBC	$3.8 \times 10^9/l$
Platelets	$154 \times 10^9/l$

   Questions:

   1. Give the two most likely diagnoses.

   2. What investigations would you arrange? Give four.

4. A 28 year old Ghanaian woman comes to the ante-natal booking clinic with her first pregnancy, last menstrual period seven weeks ago. Her booking haemoglobin is 10.9 g/dl, MCV 86 fl with normal WBC and platelets, and screening test for sickle haemoglobin is positive. Haemoglobin electrophoresis shows HbA 55%, HbS 45%. Her partner is investigated and his count and haemoglobin electrophoretic findings are as follows:

Hb	11.6 g/dl
RBC	$5.9 \times 10^{12}/l$
MCV	64 fl
HbA	band only, HbA_2 quantitation 4.2%

   Questions:

   1. What haematological diagnosis would you make for (a) the woman and (b) her partner?

   2. What conditions might the child inherit and what are their relative probabilities?

Answers overleaf

Data Interpretations : Answers

3. 1. In any patient who presents with a macrocytic anaemia, and borderline low WBC and platelet count, excessive alcohol intake is a likely diagnosis. In this man vitamin B_{12} deficiency must also be considered likely. Many strictly vegetarian or vegan Asian people develop B_{12} deficiency, as the vitamin is only present in food of animal origin.

   2. Investigations required include inspection of a blood film on which might be seen oval macrocytes and hypersegmented neutrophils in B_{12} (or folate) deficiency, and occasionally toxic effects of alcohol including vacuolation of neutrophil cytoplasm; serum B_{12} level (and folate levels if the history is suggestive), liver function tests and γ-glutamyl transferase in particular, and thyroid function tests. A bone marrow aspirate might be considered if the film or history is suggestive of myelodysplasia or myeloma, and some experts like to confirm megaloblastic erythropoiesis if B_{12} deficiency is thought to be the problem. A Schilling test should be performed if a low B_{12} level is found.

4. 1. (a) The woman has sickle cell trait, Hb AS, with no evidence of additional haemoglobinopathy (the MCV is normal, slightly more Hb A than S is normal in the trait). (b) The partner has β-thalassaemia trait, evidenced by the marginally reduced haemoglobin, much reduced MCV and high RBC count. This could also be due to α thalassaemia trait, but the raised HbA_2 (normal range <3.5%) indicates β-thalassaemia trait. In iron deficiency, one would see a much lower Hb and RBC count at this level of microcytosis.

   2. Considering the β globin genes for this couple, the mother has one normal and one sickle β gene, the father has one normal and one thalassaemic β gene. There is an equal likelihood of either β gene from each being contributed to any one offspring. Thus there is a 1:4 chance of any child of this couple having each of the following; normal adult haemoglobin only (Hb AA), sickle cell trait, β-thalassaemia trait, and sickle-β thalassaemia. The first three conditions are clearly not associated with serious problems, but the last is a true sickling syndrome which can be as severe in its manifestations as homozygous sickle cell disease.

Haematology : Data Interpretations

5. A 9 year old boy is noted to bleed excessively after operation to remove his tonsils and adenoids. There is no previous history of bleeding or relevant family history.
   His blood count and clotting screen results are:

Hb	12.3 g/dl
WBC	8.6 x 10^9/l, normal differential
Platelets	348 x 10^9/l
PT	14 (control 13 seconds)
APTT	63 (control 35 seconds)
Thrombin time	12 (control 12 seconds)
APTT 50:50 mix with normal plasma : 39 seconds	

   Further investigations show:
   Factor VIIIC level 1.12 iu/ml (normal range 0.5–1.5 iu/ml)
   Factor IX level 0.76 iu/ml (normal range 0.5–1.5 iu/ml)
   Platelet aggregation studies show normal responses to all standard stimulating agents including ristocetin.

   Questions:
   1. What causes for a bleeding tendency, which you might otherwise suspect in this young boy, are excluded by these results? Give five.
   2. What is the remaining most likely diagnosis?

6. Following emergency laparotomy for ruptured colonic diverticulum, a 73 year old man is noted to be bleeding excessively into his abdominal drain. Pre-operative FBC and clotting screen were within the normal range.
   His current count and screen are:

Hb	9.6 g/dl
MCV	92 fl
WBC	15.8 x 10^9/l, 86% neutrophils
Platelets	47 x 10^9/l
PT	20 (control 14 seconds)
APTT	56 (control 37 seconds)
Thrombin time	38 (control 12 seconds), corrected to 22 seconds with protamine sulphate, no correction with toluidine blue.

   Question:
   1. What is the most likely haematological diagnosis?

   Answers overleaf

Data Interpretations : Answers

5. 1. The normal platelet count excludes immune thrombocytopenia, which is relatively common in children. The platelet aggregation studies make a qualitative defect of platelet function unlikely: the latter are anyway uncommon. The normal aggregation response to ristocetin together with the normal Factor VIIIC levels are against a diagnosis of von Willebrand's disease, which one might wish to confirm with a ristocetin cofactor assay and/or a von Willebrand factor antigen assay. The levels of factor VIIIC and IX are both well within the normal ranges and this excludes classical haemophilia A and haemophilia B or Christmas disease as the cause of the problem.

2. The abnormality demonstrated is a long APTT. This implicates the intrinsic pathway as being at fault, common pathway and fibrinogen problems being exonerated by the normal PT and TT respectively. The extrinsic pathway is not involved (normal PT). Of the intrinsic pathway factors, VIIIC and IX are known to be normal, this leaves XI and XII deficiencies as possible causes. Factor XII deficiency does not give rise to clinical bleeding problems, indeed a paradoxical tendency to hypercoagulability can be found. Thus deficiency of factor XI (a generally mild bleeding disorder inherited as an autosomal co-dominant trait) is the most likely remaining diagnosis, and should be confirmed by specific factor XI assay.

6. 1. The abnormalities are: long PT, APTT and thrombin time, none is extreme but the thrombin time is the most abnormal. The platelet count is also low. In the setting of acute infection (most probably peritoneal infections with large bowel organisms) the diagnosis is disseminated intravascular coagulation (DIC). The thrombin time is the most sensitive index of DIC as it tests specifically the conversion of fibrinogen to fibrin by added thrombin; it is prolonged in this condition because of (a) reduced fibrinogen level secondary to consumption and (b) the presence of fibrin degradation products (FDPs), which interfere with the formation of cross-linked fibrin. Protamine sulphate, better known for its neutralisation of heparin, also corrects to a degree for FDPs; toluidine blue can correct for the dysfibrinogen of liver disease but not FDPs, so the TT remains abnormal in the presence of this reagent.

Haematology : Data Interpretations

7. A 38 year old Nigerian woman required a four unit whole blood transfusion for postpartum haemorrhage after the birth of her second child. Pre-transfusion antibody screening was clear, and the crossmatch was straightforward with no incompatibilities. Following transfusion her Hb was 11.1 g/dl.

   Six days later she was noted to be jaundiced, with the following haematology and biochemistry results:

Hb	7.9 g/dl
MCV	96 fl
Reticulocytes	4.5%
WBC	12.8 x 10^9/l, 76% neutrophils
Platelets	604 x 10^9/l
Serum bilirubin	65 µmol/l

   Direct Coombs test positive

   Questions:

   1. What do you think has happened?
   2. What investigations will you arrange to clarify the cause of the problem?

8. A 40 year old Cypriot woman was admitted to hospital for dilatation and curettage for menorrhagia.

   Her pre-operative investigations were:

Hb	10.5 g/dl
WBC	7.8 x 10^9/l
RBC	5.7 x 10^{12}/l
MCV	67 fl
MCH	18.4 pg
MCHC	24 g/dl
Platelets	402 x 10^9/l

   Questions:

   1. What are the two most likely diagnoses?
   2. Give four investigations to elucidate the diagnosis further.

   Answers overleaf

Data Interpretations : Answers

7. 1. It is likely that the woman is suffering from a delayed haemolytic transfusion reaction. This arises especially in people who have been previously transfused or in women who have been pregnant (and thus exposed to 'foreign' red cell antigens).

2. The patient's direct Coombs test (DCT) should be checked and unless all the transfused cells bearing the relevant antigen have been destroyed already, will usually be positive. The important test is to re-screen serum taken now, at re-presentation, against a panel of red cells of known phenotype in order to try and identify the antibody specificity. Antibody-formers frequently make more than one antibody so the search should not stop when one is identified. It is useful, if possible, to type the units she received to check how many of them bear the relevant antigen. As well as confirming that the reaction could have arisen at this transfusion it is useful to estimate how many of the units one could expect her to destroy.

8. 1. The two common causes of a microcytic anaemia in such a case are iron deficiency anaemia and thalassaemia trait.

2. To differentiate between these two diagnoses, the blood film may be of value, 'pencil cells' and anisocytosis in general being more marked in iron deficiency, and target cells more frequent in thalassaemia trait. The serum iron and total iron binding capacity (or ferritin if available) should be measured and may confirm iron deficiency; the serum iron, or ferritin, may be normal or even slightly high in thalassaemia trait. Haemoglobin electrophoresis at alkaline pH shows a slightly increased band of the minor adult haemoglobin HbA_2 in β-thalassaemia trait which should be quantified (normal range being <3.5% of total Hb). The HbA_2 may be falsely low in the presence of iron deficiency, so ideally the iron status should first be checked and any deficiency corrected before the HbA_2 estimation is performed. If the iron status is normal and the HbA_2 is not elevated, the blood picture should be interpreted as consistent with α-thalassaemia trait. It is not usually necessary to confirm this formally, but if needed (for example for ante-natal counselling purposes), the definitive check for α and β-thalassaemia trait is a globin chain synthesis study.

9. A 50 year old woman on drug treatment for Parkinson's disease complained of increasing shortness of breath and malaise.

Investigations showed:

Hb	8.8 g/dl
WBC	$8.1 \times 10^9/l$
RBC	$4.4 \times 10^{12}/l$
Platelets	$350 \times 10^9/l$
MCV	109 fl
MCH	26 pg
MCHC	36 g/dl
PCV	32%

Film: macrocytosis, polychromasia, spherocytes noted.

Questions:

1. What three investigations are indicated?

2. What is the cause of her raised MCV?

3. Give three possible causes of the anaemia.

Answers overleaf

9. 1. The picture of a macrocytic anaemia with a film showing polychromasia and spherocytes suggests haemolysis. Further investigations should include a direct antiglobulin test (direct Coombs test [DCT]), a reticulocyte count and a measurement of serum and red cell folate since utilisation of this vitamin is increased in haemolysis and deficiency readily occurs. Deficiency exacerbates the anaemia: a clue may be found on the blood film if hypersegmented neutrophils are seen.

2. 'Reticulocytes' (which are only seen after special supra-vital staining of the blood sample and cannot be seen on the ordinary blood film) correspond to the blue-staining polychromatic cells on the blood film, and are larger than older red cells, therefore reticulocytosis itself causes a raised MCV. Folate deficiency may be contributing to her macrocytosis.

3. The most likely cause of her anaemia is immune mediated haemolysis secondary to L-dopa treatment for her Parkinson's disease; her DCT should be positive. Like α-methyldopa, this can cause a 'true' autoimmune haemolysis, with antibody directed against antigens (frequently of rhesus specificity) on the red cell membrane. Many other drugs have been implicated in the genesis of immune haemolysis, including mefanamic acid, penicillins, and some cephalosporins. Folate deficiency may be contributing to her anaemia. Other causes of auto-immune haemolysis should be considered, (especially if she is not taking any relevant drugs), for example idiopathic immune haemolysis, connective tissue disorders (systemic lupus erythematosus, rheumatoid disease), lymphoproliferative disorders or viral infections.

Haematology : Data Interpretations

10. Three days after a laparotomy for ovarian cyst, a 38 year old woman suffers a deep venous thrombosis in the leg with evidence of localised pulmonary embolism. She is put onto a continuous intravenous infusion of heparin and after a further five days (day 8) starts on oral warfarin while continuing on the heparin infusion. She receives 10 mg on day 8 and 5 mg on day 9, and on day 10 gives the following results:

Hb	10.9 g/dl
WBC	15.6 x 10^9/l
Platelets	42 x 10^9/l
PT	38 (control 13 seconds)
APTT	108 (control 36 seconds)
TT	>100 (control 11 seconds). No correction of TT with protamine sulphate 1% in vitro, correction to 14 seconds with protamine sulphate 10% in vitro
INR	3.2

Questions:

1. Explain the findings in the full blood count.

2. Is this woman receiving too much heparin? Explain your conclusion.

3. What management do you now advise?

Answers overleaf

Data Interpretations : Answers

10. 1. Thrombocytopenia is not uncommon after heparin therapy of several days duration: It may relate to the activation of platelets by heparin with their premature removal from the circulation. However, it is usually of mild degree and a platelet count as low as $42 \times 10^9/l$ might be attributed to heparin on another basis: more rarely the drug induces heparin-mediated anti-platelet antibodies and can cause profound thrombocytopenia. This is an idiosyncratic reaction. The treatment for both kinds of thrombocytopenia is to stop the heparin. There is a suggestion that the newer low molecular weight heparins may not induce thrombocytopenia to the same extent.

2. The PT and INR are increased by the warfarin treatment she has received, and the level is within the desired therapeutic range. Heparin prolongs the APTT and the TT, it affects the PT relatively little. One can monitor heparin therapy by either of the first two tests: the APTT should be between 1.5–2 times control (about 50–80 seconds is the range frequently used), the thrombin time should be between 60–100 seconds or >100 seconds if there is correction with 1% protamine sulphate. On both these tests, therefore, this woman is receiving too much heparin.

3. The INR is now within the therapeutic range and the heparin can safely be stopped: indeed it must be stopped because of the thrombocytopenia and because she is receiving too high a dose. She has proved to be quite sensitive to warfarin, rapidly entering the therapeutic range on small loading doses, so her ultimate requirement will probably be only 3 mg or so daily. After stopping the heparin, it is hoped that the platelet count will gradually return to normal; this must be frequently monitored and she must be examined carefully for signs of bleeding in the meantime.

Haematology : Data Interpretations

11. A 55 year old Caucasian male complained of dizziness and thumping headaches. He was receiving diuretic treatment for mild hypertension. He had recently been trying to lose weight, without success, and had also unsuccessfully tried to give up smoking. His brother had recently died, aged 59, from a myocardial infarction. On examination there were signs of chronic airway obstruction but no other abnormal findings.
Investigations showed:

Hb	18.5 g/dl	MCHC	33.5 g/dl
WBC	6.5 x 10^9/l	PCV	45.5%
RBC	6.3 x 10^{12}/l	Plasma sodium	139 mmol/l
Platelets	305 x 10^9/l	potassium	3.9 mmol/l
ESR	4 mm in first hour	urea	6.5 mmol/l
MCH	29.3 pg	Serum creatinine	132 µmol/l
MCV	87 fl		

Questions:

1. What is the differential diagnosis? Give two.
2. What further investigations would you request? Suggest five.

2. A 31 year old male homosexual with AIDS presents complaining of fatigue, shortness of breath and lethargy. He has had a low grade fever (37–37.8°C) for the past 10 days. He has had a previous episode of pneumocystis pneumonia and is on maintenance Septrin together with AZT (azacytidine).
Investigations show:

Hb	6.9 g/dl
WBC	1.9 x 10^9/l, neutrophils 78%, lymphocytes 16%, monocytes 5%, eosinophils 1%
RBC	30 x 10^{12}/l
Platelets	59 x 10^9/l
MCH	21.5 pg
MCV	115 fl
MCHC	19.1 g/dl
PCV	34.5%

Questions:

1. Suggest two causes for the raised MCV.
2. Suggest three causes for his pancytopenia.

Answers overleaf

Data Interpretations : Answers

11. 1. The differential diagnosis for this man's raised Hb and PCV (i.e. polycythaemia) lies between true polycythaemia, either primary or secondary, and apparent or 'stress' polycythaemia. In the former, there is an absolute increase in red cell mass, in the latter the red cell mass is within the normal range but the plasma volume is reduced, giving rise to the increased red cell 'concentration' in the circulation.

2. These two possible diagnoses can be differentiated by isotopic measurement of red cell mass and plasma volume. If 'true' polycythaemia is discovered, this might be due to a primary marrow overproduction (polycythaemia rubra vera [PRV]) or secondary to increased erythropoietin drive (for example due to chronic hypoxia or inappropriate erythropoietin from a renal lesion). Other investigations should thus include chest X-ray (plus respiratory function tests), arterial blood gases, and renal imaging studies – ultrasound or intravenous urogram. Occasionally a high affinity haemoglobin can cause this syndrome; one might suspect this if other family members were affected and haemoglobin electrophoresis and oxygen dissociation studies of Hb might help. Stress polycythaemia is usually seen in obese middle aged male hypertensives, and diuretic therapy may contribute towards the low plasma volume. This man would be a typical candidate for this syndrome. Also in favour of this diagnosis rather than primary polycythaemia would be the normal WBC and platelet count (an element of neutrophilia and/or thrombocytosis being common in PRV) and the absence of a palpable spleen.

12. 1. AZT therapy consistently causes a macrocytosis, and folate deficiency is also frequent in AIDS patients on a dietary basis, due to chronic diarrhoea and due to Septrin treatment.

2. The anaemia might be drug induced, attributable to AZT or Septrin; the former always causes macrocytosis and commonly anaemia requiring transfusion. Less commonly other cell lines are similarly depressed. Profound folate deficiency can cause leucopenia and thrombocytopenia as well as anaemia. Immune cytopenias (with adequate marrow production but peripheral destruction of cells) of any or all cell lines can occur in AIDS. Marrow infiltration by lymphoma needs to be considered. A variety of opportunistic infections can cause depression of haematopoiesis (for example mycobacterial infection), as can viral agents such as hepatitis B and Epstein Barr virus.

RHEUMATOLOGY : CASE HISTORIES

1. A 50 year old gentleman is referred to the rheumatology clinic with a three-day history of a hot swollen right knee and no preceding trauma. He gave a four-year history of generalised polyarthralgia and a six-months history of pain and stiffness of joints. Over the six months prior to presentation he had noticed generalised malaise and weakness associated with some weight loss. He had a past history of investigation for intermittent right upper quadrant pain for which no cause could be found, and had also been counselled for impotence. Examination revealed a pigmented, thin gentleman, with bruising of the arms and bleeding of the gums. An enlarged, firm liver 5 cm below the right costal margin was noted. Tender swelling of the second and third metacarpophalangeal joints of both hands were found. A large effusion of the right knee was aspirated yielding 50 ml of turbid, straw-coloured fluid.

   Questions:
   1. What is the diagnosis?
   2. Give three tests which would be useful in the diagnosis of this condition.
   3. Explain the possible mechanisms for the abnormal bleeding.
   4. What is the cause of the mono-arthritis of the knee?

2. A 27 year old girl is seen in casualty with diplopia. She has been unwell for the preceding month with malaise and intermittent fevers with some weight loss. Over the preceding three years several episodes of polyarthralgia associated with vasculitic lesions appearing over the elbows had been treated by oral prednisolone. Five years prior to presentation she had been seen by the ENT surgeons with chronic sinusitis, and later required nasal reconstructive surgery following a nasal collapse. On examination she was pyrexial with a temperature of 39°C. Vasculitic lesions were noted over the elbows. Central nervous system examination revealed normal visual acuity in both eyes with no obvious ocular muscle weakness. The diplopia, however, was elicited on right lateral gaze. Chest X-ray on admission revealed a well-circumscribed round lesion in the right upper zone approximately 8 cm in diameter.

   Questions:
   1. What is the probable diagnosis?
   2. What three investigations may be of help in the management of this condition?

Answers overleaf

Case Histories : Answers

1.
1. Haemochromatosis.

2. The three useful tests in the diagnosis include estimation of the body serum iron stores by measurement of the serum transferrin, iron, and serum iron-binding capacity. Other tests which would give characteristic results are radiology of the hands which will reveal cystic change and sclerosis of subchondral bone with loss of articular cartilage and chondrocalcinosis, classically occurring in the second and third metacarpophalangeal joints of the hands. Liver biopsy may be indicated to assess progression to cirrhosis. Finally, HLA tissue typing reveals a marked association between primary haemochromatosis and the HLA A3 B14 gene locus.

3. The bleeding gums may be due to abnormal liver function with subsequent clotting abnormalities. However there is also an association between frank scurvy and iron overload (as found in haemochromatosis) because of the chronic depletion of ascorbic acid by accelerated oxidation to oxalic acid.

4. The mono-arthritis seen in 15–50% of patients with haemochromatosis is due to an acute pyrophosphate crystal arthritis.

2.
1. This young lady has Wegener's granulomatosis.

2. Diagnosis is often delayed by an atypical presentation with symptoms wrongly attributed to other connective tissue diseases. Unlike the latter diseases, however, the ANA is usually negative or present in low positive titre and unlike acute systemic lupus erythematosus the neutrophil count rises during attacks accompanied by a thrombocytosis, high ESR and high C-reactive protein levels. More recently auto-antibodies against neutrophil cytoplasm have been described, and in some patients are useful as an adjunct to diagnosis. Histological specimens are often unhelpful in view of the tissue necrosis. In this case a CT scan of the sinuses and orbits revealed masses in both sinuses and the right orbit.

Rheumatology : Case Histories

3. A 35 year old man is seen in the rheumatology out-patient clinic with a six-year history of intermittent arthritis affecting his knees and ankles. He gave a past history of having been investigated for intermittent, anterior chest pain and had also had intermittent diarrhoea and steatorrhoea. Examination revealed finger clubbing with subcutaneous nodules over the elbows. Small effusions were noted in both knees. Spinal examination revealed a full range of movement with no tenderness of the sacro-iliac joints. Further investigations revealed normal X-rays of the spine, pelvis and sacro-iliac joints. There was no evidence of an erosive arthritis. He was found to be positive for HLA B27 and a small bowel biopsy showed, on microscopy, an abundance of macrophages filled with PAS positive material in the lamina propria of the small intestine.

Questions:
1. What is the probable diagnosis?
2. What treatment should be given for this gentleman's arthritis?

4. A 26 year old man is seen in the rheumatology out-patient department with a one-month history of symmetrical polyarthritis affecting the interphalangeal, wrist, knee and ankle joints. He had been seen in the out-patient clinic two years previously with acute mono-arthritis of the right knee, 10 days after an episode of non-specific urethritis. During his current episode of arthritis he had noticed weight loss of approximately half a stone and he had developed, for the first time, a florid psoriaform rash over trunk, scalp and legs. On examination he was pyrexial with a temperature of 38°C, lymphadenopathy in axilla and groins was noted and mild oral candidiasis. An acute synovitis was found affecting the painful joints with moderate effusions of both knees. In view of the severity of his symptoms he was admitted to the ward for bed rest and commenced on indomethacin 75 mg b.d. Two days later he complained of feeling increasingly unwell and short of breath. A chest X-ray was unremarkable and auscultation revealed no obvious abnormality. He complained of increasing shortness of breath and over the next 24 hours became cyanosed and confused. A chest X-ray showed bilateral fine pulmonary shadowing. He was transferred to the intensive therapy unit and a Swan-Ganz catheter inserted, this revealed normal right heart and left atrial pressures.

Questions:
1. What is the underlying diagnosis?
2. What is the cause of the arthritis?
3. What investigation should now be performed?

Answers overleaf

Case Histories : Answers

3. 1. This gentleman has a sero-negative polyarthritis and the association with diarrhoea makes one of the gut associated spondyloarthropathies a likely diagnosis. The presence of PAS-positive material in macrophages on the small bowel biopsy is highly suggestive of the diagnosis of Whipple's disease. 60% of patients with this diagnosis are affected rheumatologically before their gastrointestinal symptoms appear.

2. The arthritis is not responsive to standard gold or penicillamine therapy and often settles following protracted therapy with either penicillin, erythromycin or tetracycline.

4. 1. This gentleman has HIV infection which is converting to the AIDS syndrome. Although he presents with a florid psoriaform rash and a polyarthritis suggestive of psoriatic arthritis the unusual feature in the history is the lack of preceding history of psoriasis. Although both lymphadenopathy and pyrexia can be seen with acute psoriatic arthritis oral candidiasis is unusual. Furthermore he has a past history of a sexually transmitted disease followed by a reactive arthritis.

2. Development of a psoriatic arthritis de novo in patients with previously asymptomatic HIV infection and their subsequent deterioration has been reported. Furthermore, this gentleman then developed shortness of breath whilst taking indomethacin. Although this could be due to asthma induced by the non-steroidal agent or to pulmonary oedema as an idiosyncratic response, it was in fact due to pneumocystis infection which is often difficult to detect early by chest X-ray.

3. To confirm the diagnosis, his HIV antibody status and antigen status should be checked.

Rheumatology : Case Histories

5. A 56 year old man contacted rheumatology out-patients, complaining of a one-week history of intermittent diplopia. He had been under the care of the department for five years with sero-positive erosive nodular rheumatoid arthritis. Over the past six months his arthritis had been active and he had been started on indomethacin 75 mg b.d. and D-penicillamine 750 mg daily. He had a past history of thyrotoxicosis treated with radio-iodine and was currently taking thyroxine replacement 0.2 mg daily. He was found to have relatively quiescent rheumatoid arthritis and neurological examination was unremarkable except mild weakness of the upper limbs was noted.

Questions:

1. What are the two most likely diagnoses in this man?

2. What two further investigations may be helpful in managing this patient?

6. A 48 year old lady with longstanding seropositive rheumatoid arthritis contacted her GP complaining of a two-day history of increasing shortness of breath. Her medication at the time was indomethacin 75 mg b.d. and methotrexate 7.5 mg once weekly commenced one week previously. Prior to this she had been receiving intramuscular gold 50 mg six-weekly. This had been discontinued due to lack of effect one month earlier. On examination her temperature was 36.6°C, blood pressure 110/70 mm Hg, JVP was not elevated and mild bilateral ankle oedema was noted. Examination of the respiratory system revealed tachypnoea with bilateral fine crepitations. An active synovitis of wrists and knees was noted. An ECG was unremarkable.

Question:

1. Give three possible diagnoses.

Answers overleaf

Case Histories : Answers

5. 1. Diplopia with rheumatoid arthritis is unusual. Occasionally it may be due to tenosynovitis affecting the tendon of the superior oblique muscle and occasionally vasculitis. This patient however has developed myasthenia and the question to be answered is whether this is secondary to his penicillamine therapy or primary myasthenia gravis.

2. HLA tissue typing has been found to be of help in distinguishing between these two conditions. There is an increased prevalence of HLA BW 35 and DR1 in patients with drug induced myasthenia gravis, in contrast to patients with spontaneous myasthenia gravis who often have the HLA B8 DR3 locus. EMG studies and a tensilon test should also be carried out to confirm the diagnosis.

6. 1. Pulmonary complications are relatively common in rheumatoid arthritis (RA), with pneumonia accounting for the majority of deaths. The rapidly increasing shortness of breath over two weeks with bilateral crepitations in this patient could be due to pneumonia secondary to immunosuppression with methotrexate – though the dose is small and she had only just started the drug. Pulmonary fibrosis occurs in RA but would be unlikely to present acutely. Similarly left ventricular failure is a possibility though unlikely in view of the patient's age and sex. A pneumonitis secondary to methotrexate is a possibility and can occur even after a single dose.

RHEUMATOLOGY : DATA INTERPRETATIONS

1. A 28 year old woman with a past history of butterfly rashes and polyarthralgia is referred by the obstetric department. Aged 21 years she had a DVT whilst on the contraceptive pill and since has had three miscarriages at 16–18 weeks and a recent intra-uterine death (IUD) at 30 weeks. Following the recent IUD she developed an extensive femoral vein thrombosis.
   Investigations showed:

   Hb 11 g/dl
   WBC 6.0×10^9/l, normal differential
   Platelets 40×10^9/l
   Creatinine clearance 120 ml/minute
   ANA 1 in 40
   ENA negative
   DNA crithidia positive 1 in 10
   VDRL positive 1 in 1
   Plasma sodium 140 mmol/l
   potassium 4.2 mmol/l
   urea 4.0 mmol/l

   Questions:
   1. What is the diagnosis?
   2. What further tests should be done?
   3. What precautions should be advised in subsequent pregnancies?

2. A 23 year old man is seen in the neurology out-patients department with an eight-week history of malaise and migratory pains in muscles and joints, persistent headaches and a recent left seventh nerve palsy. Two months prior to his presentation he returned from a camping holiday in America and had developed a generalised annular rash over his trunk, which had settled without treatment. Over the week prior to his attendance in the neurology out-patients, he noticed pain and swelling of the left knee.
   Investigations showed:

   Hb 11 g/dl
   WBC 6.0×10^9/l
   ESR 50 mm in the first hour
   Rheumatoid factor negative
   Antinuclear antibody negative
   Biochemical profile normal

   Questions:
   1. What is the diagnosis?
   2. What confirmatory test should be carried out?

Answers overleaf

Data Interpretations : Answers

1. 1. This patient has systemic lupus erythematosus by the revised American Rheumatology Association criteria.

2. The combination of recurrent thrombosis, miscarriage and thrombocytopenia is suggestive of the antiphospholipid syndrome. The VDRL is positive with neat serum (suggestive of the biological false positive test). Other tests which should be done include the lupus anticoagulant which involves the in vitro demonstration of prolongation of phospholipid dependent clotting studies which do not correct with the addition of normal plasma. The antiphospholipid antibodies may also be demonstrated by an anticardiolipin ELISA.

3. In future pregnancies the patient will require anticoagulation to prevent further thromboses. Due to the teratogenicity of warfarin subcutaneous heparin is advisable for at least the first trimester, with conversion back from warfarin if used, to heparin in the weeks prior to delivery. The causes of the fetal losses seen in such women are currently under investigation as are therapies. At present a combination of heparin, low dose aspirin, and steroids are being used on a trial basis.

2. 1. The diagnosis is Lyme disease. Early in the illness many patients suffer malaise and musculoskeletal pain. 15% of patients develop frank neurological abnormalities of which facial palsy is relatively common.

2. The confirmatory test is an antibody titre directed against *Borrelia burgdorferi* and treatment is with antibiotics.

Rheumatology : Data Interpretations

3. A 24 year old man is seen in casualty complaining of a painful right knee. He had previously been brought to the casualty department on several occasions and was known to be living rough with several other young squatters in a derelict Victorian house. On examination he appeared pale, thin and disorientated in time and space. On examination the right knee was hot and swollen. Examination was otherwise unhelpful and there were no focal neurological signs. The fundi appeared normal.

Investigations on admission:

Hb	8 g/dl
WBC	4.1×10^9/l
Platelets	200×10^9/l
Plasma sodium	140 mmol/l
potassium	5.0 mmol/l
urea	25 mmol/l
Serum creatinine	300 µmol/l
uric acid	1.6 mmol/l
calcium	2.2 mmol/l
albumin	36 g/l
total protein	80 g/l

Blood film revealed basophilic stippling of the red cells.

Joint aspirate: 20,000 polymorphs/ml; no organisms seen; intracellular negatively birefringent crystals detected.

Questions:

1. What is the diagnosis?

2. What is the underlying cause?

Answers overleaf

Data Interpretations : Answers

3. 1. This young man has acute gout affecting the right knee. There is no history of alcohol abuse. His biochemical profile is suggestive of renal impairment, though the uric acid is markedly elevated. He is also anaemic with basophilic stippling. This combination is suggestive of renal impairment secondary to heavy metal poisoning with lead and the subsequent development of saturnine gout.

2. Lead may be ingested in large quantities by people living in old Victorian buildings where lead paint may have been used on wood surfaces and may also be acquired in quantities by drinking water from lead pipes commonly found in these houses. The initial disorientation was due to an encephalopathy induced by the lead poisoning which reversed following treatment.

Rheumatology : Data Interpretations

4. A 67 year old man is seen in the casualty department with a two-day history of fever and retrosternal pain. Approximately six months prior to his admission he had been admitted to hospital with a myocardial infarction and subsequently had received atenolol 100 mg daily and hydralazine 50 mg t.d.s. for hypertension. Over the three months prior to being seen in casualty he developed pains in his hands and shoulders.

Investigations showed:

Hb	11.0 g/dl
WBC	$4.0 \times 10^9/l$
Platelets	$250 \times 10^9/l$

Rheumatoid factor negative
Anti-nuclear antibodies 1 in 320
ECG revealed elevation of the ST segments in all leads
Cardiac enzymes: normal

Questions:

1. What is the likely diagnosis?

2. Give two blood tests which would be helpful in making the diagnosis?

Answers overleaf

Data Interpretations : Answers

4. 1. This patient is suffering from a drug induced lupus syndrome presenting with arthralgia and pericarditis. The features which are suggestive are the patient's age and his on-going therapy with both atenolol and hydralazine, although the latter is much more commonly associated with the syndrome.

2. Useful tests would include measurement of the DNA and ENA antibodies which in a drug induced syndrome are usually negative. Anti-histone antibodies can also be assayed which are more characteristically positive in drug induced lupus.

5. A previously fit 24 year old girl is referred from the Obstetric Department. She is 10 weeks pregnant with her first child. From the eighth week of pregnancy she developed joint pains and over the preceding week her weight has increased by 2 kg.

On examination moderate pitting oedema is noted with the JVP elevated 2 cm. The BP is 180/120 mm Hg and a 3rd heart sound is noted. Fundoscopy reveals two cotton wool spots.

Investigations showed:

Hb	11.0 g/dl
WBC	3.2 x 10^9/l, lymphocytes 0.2 x 10^9/l
Platelets	40 x 10^9/l
ESR	120 mm in the first hour

Antinuclear antibody	1 in 160
DNA	crithidia positive 1 in 10
Complement	C4 low

Urine blood	+++
protein	+++
Urinary microscopy	granular casts ++

Plasma	sodium	140 mmol/l
	potassium	5.6 mmol/l
	urea	20 mmol/l
Serum	creatinine	200 µmol/l
	total protein	50 g/l
	albumin	16 g/l

Questions:

1. What is the diagnosis?

2. How would you manage this patient?

3. What advice would you give about subsequent pregnancies?

Answers overleaf

Data Interpretations : Answers

5. 1. This patient presents with an acute glomerulonephritis in early pregnancy. The features include fluid overload, hypertension, mild hyperkalaemia and nephrotic syndrome. The low platelet count, relative lymphopaenia, low C4 and positive ANA and DNA antibodies are suggestive that the nephritis is secondary to systemic lupus erythematosus.

   2. Management involves:

      a) Control of the hypertension. Although vasodilators are the first preference, combination therapy is often required.

      b) Reduction of potassium levels.

      c) Achievement of fluid balance.

      d) Treatment of the underlying nephritis. Renal biopsy is indicated.

      e) The effects of these therapies on the fetus should be considered and if an aggressive nephritis is found termination of the pregnancy is a major consideration in view of the poor prognosis for both mother and fetus.

   3. Early treatment of the nephritis results in the preservation of renal function in the majority of patients. If the nephritis is in remission future pregnancy is not contraindicated but immunosuppressant therapy (for example azathioprine) may be required. Careful monitoring of mother and fetus is therefore essential.

Rheumatology : Data Interpretations

6. A 23 year old West Indian girl presents with a flitting arthritis affecting proximal interphalangeal joints, knees and ankles, which had been present for three weeks prior to her presentation. She also has noticed tender red nodules over the anterior surfaces of both shins and a feeling of malaise.

Investigations showed:

Hb	11.0 g/dl
WBC	15.0 x 10^9/l
ESR	90 mm in the first hour
ASO	titre <200
ANA	1 in 10
ENA	negative

Rheumatoid factor 1:40

Plasma	sodium	140 mmol/l
	potassium	4.0 mmol/l
	urea	6.0 mmol/l
Serum	urate	0.62 mmol/l

X-rays of the hand showed soft tissue swelling around the proximal interphalangeal joints.
Chest X-ray showed bilateral hilar lymphadenopathy.

Question:

1. What is the diagnosis?

Answers overleaf

Data Interpretations : Answers

6. 1. The diagnosis is acute sarcoid arthritis (Lofgrens syndrome). Hyperuricaemia is found in approximately 25% of patients with acute sarcoidosis and rheumatoid factor is present in approximately 15% of patients. In this form of arthritis synovial effusions are relatively uncommon.

7. A 50 year old woman presents with a two-year history of a purpuric rash on the lower legs, worse on exercise, and mild polyarthralgia. Over the six months prior to presentation she has become increasingly weak. Examination reveals parotid enlargement and a global muscle weakness. The Schirmer test is dry.

Initial investigations showed:

Hb	11.0 g/dl
WBC	6.2×10^9/l
Platelets	400×10^9/l
ESR	90 mm in first hour

ANA	negative
Rheumatoid factor	>1:5000
Bone marrow	normal

Plasma	sodium	130 mmol/l
	potassium	2.2 mmol/l
	urea	6.0 mmol/l
Serum	total protein	130 g/l

Questions:

1. What is the diagnosis?

2. What other immunological tests may be helpful?

3. Why is the patient weak?

Data Interpretations : Answers

7. 1. This woman has Sjogren's syndrome. Other possible diagnoses include hyperglobulinaemia purpura secondary to myeloma though the normal marrow and peripheral blood film are against this.

2. Other immunological tests which could be helpful are the ENA antibody profile which gives a positive Ro in most patients with Sjogren's, and an estimation of circulating immune complexes.

3. The patient's weakness could be due to hypokalaemia, osteomalacia secondary to a renal tubular acidosis, or the peripheral neuropathy which may occur in patients with Sjogren's.

8. A 23 year old woman is referred to the rheumatology department by the general medical team. She has been extensively investigated for a six-months history of pyrexia of unknown origin (PUO). The fever originally commenced following an episode of tonsillitis and throughout the six months she had been seen she had recurrent sore throats. She had a daily fever of approximately 39°C, associated with a pink macular rash over the trunk and arms which faded as the fever settled in the morning. She also had intermittent episodes of pleurisy and over the two weeks prior to her referral had developed severe neck pain and bilateral wrist synovitis. On examination she was pyrexial with a temperature of 39.5°C, her spleen was palpable two fingers below the left costal margin. A pericardial rub was audible. Bilateral synovitis of the wrists was noted.

Investigations showed:

Hb 9.0 g/dl
WBC 24 x 10^9/l, 95% neutrophils
ESR 100 mm in first hour

Rheumatoid factor negative
Antinuclear antibody negative
ENA negative
DNA negative
Chest X-ray unremarkable
Echocardiogram small pericardial effusion

Questions:

1. What is the most likely diagnosis?

2. What treatment would you recommend?

Data Interpretations : Answers

8. 1. This patient presents with a typical history of adult onset Still's disease. Investigation of PUO and joint pains is centred primarily towards excluding infective causes or underlying malignancy such as lymphoma. The diagnosis of adult Still's is often therefore delayed.

   2. Treatment is difficult. However, benefit is often gained by the patient taking aspirin. Acute attacks of pericarditis and pleurisy may be helped by systemic steroids.

9. A 72 year old man presents with severe back pain radiating down the right leg. He has otherwise been relatively fit and well and the pain has come on over a period of two weeks though he could not remember a precipitating injury.

Investigations showed:

Hb	13.0 g/dl
WBC	6.0 x 10^9/l
ESR	10 mm in the first hour

Plasma	sodium	140 mmol/l
	potassium	4.2 mmol/l
	creatinine	140 µmol/l
	urea	9.0 mmol/l
Serum	calcium	2.3 mmol/l
	phosphate	1.2 mmol/l
	alkaline phosphatase	1500 iu/l

An X-ray of the lumbar spine revealed increased density around the edges of the vertebral bodies giving a picture frame appearance, and multiple large osteophytes. A bone scan revealed increased activity in lumbar vertebrae four and five with hot lesions in the left hemi-pelvis and right femur.

Question:

1. What is the diagnosis?

Data Interpretations : Answers

9. 1. The probable diagnosis in this patient with a disproportionately elevated alkaline phosphatase in the face of normal serum calcium and phosphate and the classical picture frame appearance of the vertebrae is Paget's disease. The cause of the pain may be referred pain from the spine though fractures are not uncommon and also nerve entrapment may occur due to bony distortion.

Rheumatology : Data Interpretations

0. A 43 year old woman presents with a two-months history of aching in her arms and legs with progressive weakness. During her illness she has noticed weight loss of approximately 1 stone and a rash worse after sunbathing over the dorsum of both arms and of her neck. On examination a purple discolouration is noted round both eyes, and the nail beds of the fingers of both hands appear erythematous.

Initial investigations showed:

Hb	10.0 g/dl
WBC	34.0 x 10^9/l, neutrophils 28.4 x 10^9/l, lymphocytes 1.8 x 10^9/l
Platelets	255 x 10^9/l
ESR	50 mm in the first hour

Plasma	sodium	136 mmol/l
	potassium	4.8 mmol/l
	urea	8.7 mmol/l
Serum	albumin	24 g/l
	globulin	29 g/l
	IgG	12.6 g/l (normal range 5.3–16.5)
	IgA	2.2 g/l (normal range 0.8–4.0)
	IgM	2.0 g/l (normal range 0.5–2.0)
	total protein	53 g/l
	creatine phosphokinase	3,800 iu/l
	aspartate transaminase	192 iu/l
	alphahydroxybutyrate dehydrogenase	955 iu/l

An EMG examination of the right deltoid muscle showed profuse spontaneous activity and small polyphasic units. Severe changes were found in the right vastus medialis muscle.

Questions:

1. What is the diagnosis?

2. What five other investigations should be performed?

Answers overleaf

Data Interpretations : Answers

10. 1. The diagnosis is dermatomyositis. This, occurring in a middle aged woman, should be investigated for an underlying malignant disease although the incidence of malignancy is low and in most cases investigation is negative.

2. For a woman the usual screening would be a biochemical profile, liver function tests, chest X-ray and pelvic examination for gynaecological malignancy. Lastly faecal occult blood should be checked and, if positive, gastroscopy and sigmoidoscopy are indicated.

Rheumatology : Data Interpretations

1. A 65 year old lady is seen in the rheumatology out-patient department complaining of aching from her cervical spine to her lower dorsal spine for approximately one year, associated with 30 minutes of early morning stiffness. Over the three months prior to her presentation she had noticed bruising of both lower legs.

Investigations showed:

Hb	9.0 g/dl
WBC	4.0 x 10^9/l
Platelets	200 x 10^9/l
ESR	120 mm in the first hour

Plasma	sodium	140 mmol/l
	potassium	4.9 mmol/l
	urea	15 mmol/l
Serum	creatinine	250 µmol/l
	calcium	3.1 mmol/l
	phosphate	2.2 mmol/l
	alkaline phosphatase	60 iu/l
	aspartate transaminase	30 iu/l
	bilirubin	6 µmol/l

Protein electrophoresis showed a global reduction in all immunoglobulins.
X-ray of the cervical and thoracic spine showed generalised osteoporosis.
Bone scan normal.

Questions:

1. What is the diagnosis?

2. What confirmatory test should be performed?

Answers overleaf

Data Interpretations : Answers

11. 1. This lady has presented with an osteoporotic spine but with the abnormal features of an elevated ESR of 120 and a raised serum calcium and phosphate with a normal alkaline phosphatase level and mild renal impairment. This suggests a diagnosis of multiple myelomatosis.

2. Multiple myeloma can be confirmed by a bone marrow examination in the majority of cases and also examination of the urine for Bence Jones proteins. Although the stiffness in the morning is suggestive of an inflammatory condition and the raised ESR suggestive of polymyalgia rheumatica, the biochemical findings are inconsistent with these diagnoses.

2.

A 65 year old man is seen in out-patients with a six-week history of severe left arm pain. The pain prevents him lying on the affected side and radiates from approximately the region of the deltoid insertion to the wrist. Apart from Moduretic for mild hypertension he is on no medication. On examination neck movements show a reduction of lateral flexion only. The left shoulder abducts to 75°, internally rotates to 25° and externally rotates to 15°.

Investigations showed:

Hb	14.5 g/dl
WBC	4.0 x 10^9/l
Platelets	239 x 10^9/l
ESR	20 mm in first hour
Blood glucose	13.8 mmol/l
Urine glucose	++

Plasma	sodium	140 mmol/l
	potassium	4.0 mmol/l
Serum	calcium	2.75 mmol/l
	urate	0.54 mmol/l
	alkaline phosphatase	112 iu/l

Question:

1. What is the diagnosis?

Answers overleaf

12. 1. This man has a capsular pattern of shoulder restriction lasting six weeks. The most likely diagnosis is adhesive capsulitis (frozen shoulder) which is associated with diabetes. Gout is very unusual in the shoulder and pain lasting six weeks would be atypical. The raised urate and calcium levels are more probably a reflection of his diuretic therapy, the need for which should be reviewed.

Rheumatology : Data Interpretations

13. A 57 year old man presents with a three-months history of pain and swelling of the third proximal interphalangeal joint of the left hand. He is otherwise fit and well, and on no medication. Although he is an accounts clerk and is right handed, the swelling has not prevented him working or pursuing his hobby of gardening. General examination is unremarkable. The left third interphalangeal joint has a flexion deformity of 5° with a range of 5–15°. There is a boggy swelling of the joint which is also noted to be warm.

Investigations showed:

Hb	13.5 g/dl
WBC	4.0 x 10^9/l
Platelets	325 x 10^9/l
ESR	25 mm in first hour
Serum calcium	2.45 mmol/l
potassium	1.1 mmol/l
urate	0.24 mmol/l
Rheumatoid factor	1 in 4 (Rose-Waaler)
ANA	negative

X-ray of the finger: soft tissue swelling noted around the joint, and loss of joint space with erosion of the margins of the joint.

Questions:

1. What would your next investigation be?
2. What is the most likely diagnosis?

14. A 24 year old physiotherapy student presents with a three-year history of intermittent low back pain lasting 3–4 days with no radiation to the legs. The only past history of note was intermittent knee pains as a teenager diagnosed as patellar subluxation. On examination the blood pressure was normal and a soft late systolic apical murmur was heard. Spinal movements were full and painless, the patient being able to put both hands flat on the floor on forward flexion. Straight leg raise was to 170° bilaterally. The reflexes in the limbs were present and symmetrical. Sensation in the legs was normal.

Questions:

1. What is the diagnosis?
2. What other joints should be examined to confirm the diagnosis?

Answers overleaf

Data Interpretations : Answers

13. 1. This gentleman presents with a mono-arthritis of the finger. Although psoriatic arthritis and reactive arthritis may present in this way there are no findings on examination to support the former or history for the latter. In any mono-arthritis local infection or trauma should be considered and it is one instance where synovial biopsy is indicated.

   2. In this case the biopsy revealed a rose thorn in the synovium which had caused the resulting synovitis. Occasionally rose thorn arthritis may result in a symmetrical polyarthritis if removal of the thorn is delayed.

14. 1. Hypermobility syndrome. The patient has intermittent back pain with evidence of hypermobility - a hypermobile spine, possible mitral valve prolapse and a past history of knee pains.

   2. Other joint abnormalities which should be sought include:

      a) Passive approximation of thumb to forearm with wrist flexion.

      b) Passive hyperextension of the digits.

      c) Active hyperextension of the knee to more than 10°.

      d) Active hyperextension of the elbow to more than 10°.

      e) Passive and excessive hyperextension of the foot and ankle and eversion of the foot.

      The diagnosis is made when three of the six features above are present.

NEUROLOGY : CASE HISTORIES

1. A 70 year old man is seen in the accident department with a mild left hemiparesis. He has a history of mild hypertension treated with a diuretic and is known to have mild angina pectoris from ischaemic heart disease. Three weeks previously, his general practitioner was called to see him because he had become unrousable. He had recovered by the time the GP saw him and had no signs. Since then his wife says that he complains of a slight left sided weakness and 'difficulty walking'.

    On initial examination the man is alert although a little vague in his history, blood pressure 200/120 and soft bilateral carotid bruits. There is no papilloedema. The only signs are a mild left sided limb weakness, in a pyramidal pattern, with bilateral extensor plantar responses. Within half an hour of his first examination, whilst having a chest X-ray in the accident department, the patient is observed to have become very drowsy. However, within fifteen minutes, when examined again, he is once more alert and there is no change in his signs.

    Questions:

    1. What is the differential diagnosis? Give five possible diagnoses.

    2. What investigations are indicated? Give two.

    3. What initial treatment should be started?

Answers overleaf

Case Histories : Answers

1. 1. The variable level of consciousness associated with only mild focal signs points to a compressive mass lesion rather than an intrinsic vascular lesion (stroke) despite the presence of vascular risk factors. The most likely diagnosis is a subdural haematoma. At least 50% of patients with chronic subdural haematoma occur without a history of trauma. High blood pressure is of course a common incidental finding and carotid bruits are coincidental findings in about 5% of elderly patients. Primary or secondary tumours are additional possible diagnoses. Obstructive hydrocephalus due to posterior fossa mass might produce the above clinical picture, though in the latter case one would expect ataxia. The absence of papilloedema cannot exclude any cause of raised intracranial pressure. Viral encephalitis is a possible diagnosis, although the level of consciousness is unlikely to be so variable, nor the course so long. An outside possibility within the differential diagnosis is a progressive carotid stenosis, although it would be unusual for this to cause the strikingly intermittent depression of conscious level with only slight focal signs shown by this patient.

2. X-ray CT scan of the head should distinguish between the above diagnoses. Since neurosurgery may be life saving in the event of a subdural haematoma a CT scan should be performed as an emergency. If the CT reveals a solitary tumour, consideration needs to be given to obtaining histology by biopsy but, first, chest X-ray should be checked for the presence of a clinically silent primary tumour. If the CT scan is normal, an EEG should be performed and the spinal fluid should be examined to exclude viral encephalitis.

3. If a mass lesion is identified the initial therapy should be directed towards reducing the intracranial pressure whilst preparations are made for more definitive neurosurgical therapy. This would be best done using dexamethasone, by injection initially. Infusion of mannitol would be indicated if the patients condition is deteriorating quickly. Subdural haematoma usually needs evacuation via cranial burr holes. However, if there is no disturbance of conscious level or focal signs, subdural haematomata is sometimes managed expectantly unless there is marked shift of intracranial contents on the CT scan.

A right handed single company representative aged 32 years, is seen in the out-patient department with a history of two blackouts. Neither of these events have been witnessed. He describes a strange feeling coming over him rather rapidly, on one of the occasions accompanied by a strange taste in his mouth. There followed a period of unconsciousness, after which he woke up feeling drowsy and when he tried to make a telephone call found that he could not speak properly. Over the next half an hour the speech disorder resolved and he had no further symptoms except on the last occasion he noted that his tongue was a bit sore. On examination there were no physical signs.

Questions:

1. What are the possible causes of this man's illness?

2. What investigations are indicated? Give three.

3. What should this man be told about his driving?

4. What treatment should be started?

Answers overleaf

Case Histories: Answers

2. 1. The most likely cause is generalised seizures, probably partial (uncal) seizures becoming secondarily generalised. The speech disorder in a right handed person indicates the focus is in the left cerebral hemisphere. The focal nature of the epilepsy increases the chances of there being an underlying structural lesion. The latter might include meningioma, glioma or metastases in or near the uncus of the temporal lobe. Infective lesions such as bacterial abscess or viral encephalitis are unlikely in the absence of pyrexia, focal deficit or alteration in conscious level. If there is immunosuppression (for example if HIV positive) toxoplasmosis may present with seizures and few or no focal signs. Even without a history of febrile convulsions in childhood mesial temporal sclerosis may cause temporal lobe epilepsy, although one would expect the presentation to have been at an earlier age.

2. Investigations required include EEG to demonstrate a focal temporal lobe abnormality and an X-ray CT scan which will identify any structural lesion. If the CT scan is normal and the EEG strongly focal, a Magnetic Resonance (MRI) scan may show mesial temporal sclerosis or other minor structural lesion.

3. The DVLC requires someone who has more than one seizure (of any degree of severity) to cease driving until they have been seizure-free for two years. The exception is if all the seizures have been during sleep and this pattern has been present for at least three years, in which case driving can continue even if the attacks persist. After a single seizure driving is usually banned for one year since the chances of recurrent seizures are maximal during that first year.

4. The best anticonvulsant for partial seizures with secondary generalisation is carbamazepine which should be started if seizures are sufficiently frequent to be causing a problem. Phenytoin is a reasonable alternative.

Neurology : Case Histories

3. A man of 19 years is seen in the accident department with a history of five days pain and weakness in his legs. About one week previously he had a flu-like illness with aching in his muscles and coryza. Over the previous five days he had developed slight drooping of his left eyelid and quite severe pain in his leg muscles, not clearly localised, and weakness of his legs with difficulty standing. On direct questioning he admitted also to some tingling in his fingers.

On examination there was a moderate left sided ptosis, slight bilateral facial weakness but otherwise normal cranial nerve function. In the limbs there was moderate weakness in upper and lower limbs more pronounced distally than proximally. Sensation to clinical testing was normal. Only the left biceps reflex was obtainable without reinforcement and the reflexes in the lower limbs were unobtainable.

Questions:

1. What are the causes of this presenting history?

2. What investigations are necessary for the diagnosis to be established?

3. What investigations are needed in the subsequent management of this disorder?

4. Is there any specific mode of therapy available in this condition?

5. What is the prognosis?

Answers overleaf

Case Histories : Answers

3. 1. The differential diagnosis is between Guillain-Barré syndrome (acute idiopathic polyradiculopathy) and myasthenia gravis. Rarer causes include poisoning with lead, thallium and botulism and acute intermittent porphyria. The loss of reflexes make the Guillain-Barré syndrome more likely than myasthenia, as does the history of sensory symptoms. Lead poisoning usually presents with a more asymmetric, multifocal predominantly motor neuropathy (wrist drop). Thallium poisoning is rare and associated with hair loss. Botulism is usually associated with marked dysautonomic features, especially dilated pupils. Porphyrins can be estimated in the blood or urine.

2. Investigations should include a Tensilon test to exclude myasthenia gravis, and a lumbar puncture. In Guillain-Barré syndrome after a few days CSF protein is raised without pleocytosis. Later, nerve conduction studies may show evidence of a demyelinating peripheral neuropathy but these tests may be normal in the early stages.

3. A crucial investigation is the early assessment of ventilatory function by measurement of the vital capacity (not peak flow). Assisted ventilation is likely once the vital capacity falls below one litre but may be needed earlier if the airway has to be protected due to severe bulbar palsy.

4. If the Guillain-Barré syndrome produces rapid disability plasmapheresis may be considered since this has been shown to reduce the period of dependency.

5. 80% of patients with Guillain-Barré syndrome achieve full functional recovery, 10% die and 10% remain disabled. Adverse prognostic features include becoming bed or chair bound within four days, advanced age and very reduced motor action potential amplitude on neurophysiological testing.

Neurology : Case Histories

4. A mother of two, aged 43 years is admitted with a weak right leg. This developed quite suddenly, though it took some days to evolve to its maximum extent. Initially there was a tendency for the foot to catch on the ground and this was accompanied by a feeling of heaviness in that limb. At the same time the patient had noticed some urgency of micturition. She had noticed no problem with the left leg or any other symptoms. A few years previously she remembered having an episode of vertigo, lasting some weeks, which had been diagnosed as vestibular neuronitis.

On examination, the only abnormality in the cranial nerves was some slowness of adduction in the right eye on rapid gaze to the left. The upper limbs were normal. In the lower limbs there was moderate weakness of hip and knee flexion, normal extension, brisk reflexes bilaterally with bilateral extensor plantar responses. There was slight diminution of joint position sense in the right great toe.

Questions:

1. What investigations should be performed? Give three.

2. What therapy might be offered?

3. Is there a risk of this woman's children having the same trouble?

Answers overleaf

Case Histories : Answers

4. 1. The first consideration should be for a myelogram to exclude a compressive lesion of the spinal cord, due to a neurofibroma or meningioma or a breast cancer metastasis for example. Back pain could be expected in the latter case. At myelography cerebrospinal fluid will be available and if the myelogram is normal the presence of a slight lymphocyte pleocytosis (less than 50/mm^3) would support the diagnosis of demyelination as would the presence of oligoclonal bands on CSF electrophoresis. Visual evoked responses will allow the detection of a previously symptomless optic neuritis and so evidence of lesions disseminated in space and time. A magnetic resonance scan would confirm the presence of other lesions in the brainstem or hemispheres caused by multiple sclerosis.

2. If significant disability is present from a demyelination cord lesion, high dose intravenous methylprednisolone speeds up recovery and improves spasticity.

3. There is a familial tendency in multiple sclerosis such that if a person has a first degree relative with the disease this increases the chances of developing the disease by between five and fifteen fold, although this risk is greater for siblings than parents.

Neurology : Case Histories

5. A 50 year old widow attended out-patients with a history of walking difficulty. For a year or so she had noticed a mild aching discomfort between her shoulder blades, somewhat worse when lying compared with standing. Over the last few months she had noticed 'stiffness' of her lower limbs and difficulty walking such that her legs were 'slowed up' and she noticed an increasing tendency to trip over uneven paving stones. Over the last few weeks she had noticed some numbness in her left lower limb and a tight feeling over her right costal margin. Some years previously she had been treated for 'sciatica' with bed rest.

On examination, cranial nerves and upper limbs were normal. There was an indefinite diminution to pinprick sensation in the left lower limb as far as the groin. There was some weakness bilaterally of hip flexion, worse on the right. There were brisk reflexes except the right ankle reflex which was absent. Plantar responses were bilaterally extensor.

Questions:

1. What investigation should be carried out?

2. What is the differential diagnosis?

3. What is the prognosis for functional recovery?

Answers overleaf

Case Histories : Answers

5. 1. The first investigation that should be performed is a myelogram. The history and signs are of a spinal cord lesion and the dull back ache makes it likely that this is at the thoracic level as does the tight radicular discomfort at the costal margin. The presence of sensory symptoms in the leg contralateral to the weaker leg suggests the Brown-Sequard syndrome of compressive myelopathy. The presence of urinary symptoms suggests that the need for investigation is becoming urgent. The absent ankle reflex can be assumed to be due to the previous sciatica presumably caused by compression of the S1 root. It may, however, be due to the presence of a second recent lesion rather than the old prolapsed disc.

2. The differential diagnosis is between a benign lesion such as a meningioma or neurofibroma (together accounting for 55% of all spinal tumours) or a malignant lesion such as a myeloma or secondary tumour from the breast or lung. A prolapsed thoracic intervertebral disc is rare and is usually accompanied by a more sudden pain. Intramedullary primary gliomas are rare and intramedullary secondary neoplasms extremely uncommon. A demyelinating myelopathy may present in a slowly progressive form at this age but would be painless. Spinal cord angioma can present with a cord compressive picture but are unusual.

3. So long as a benign compressive lesion is found (such as a meningioma, the most likely diagnosis here) and removed before bladder function is lost, a good recovery can be expected.

Neurology : Case Histories

A woman of 28 years of age comes to the accident department complaining of double vision and slight dysarthria. She describes herself as being fit and well until a few weeks ago when one evening she noticed transient diplopia, which had resolved by the next morning. Over the last few weeks this intermittent diplopia had become more pronounced and she had noticed some slurring of her words whilst talking on the telephone to her mother on the evening before presentation. Over the last year she had woken up in the middle of the night on occasions with numb fingers. There was no other history.

On examination there was variable left-sided ptosis. On testing the eye movements, there was rather variable slowness of adduction of the left eye on right gaze and diplopia which widened progressively when gazing to the right. There were no bulbar signs. Examination of the limbs showed some weakness of the pelvic girdle muscles, but reflexes were normal. In the right hand there was slight weakness and some thinning of the thenar muscles and some rather indistinct loss of pin prick over the thumb and part of the forefinger.

Questions:

1. What diagnoses would you entertain in this case? Give two.

2. What investigation(s) would you perform? Give two.

3. What therapy would be recommended assuming your principal diagnosis is correct?

Answers overleaf

Case Histories : Answers

6. 1. The two likely diagnoses are myasthenia gravis combined with median nerve compression at the carpal tunnel. The worsening of the symptoms in the evening is typical of myasthenia. The eye movements of patients with mysathenia may be confusing and, as in this case, mimic complex problems such as gaze palsies or internuclear ophthalmoplegia. The carpal tunnel syndrome provokes sensory disturbances in the thumb, forefinger and lateral aspect of the great finger, particularly at night when body fluids are redistributed away from the lower extremities. There may be weakness and wasting of muscles supplied by the median nerve, in particular the abductor pollicus brevis, producing partial thenar atrophy.

2. The initial investigation for myasthenia is a Tensilon test. 10 mg of edrophonium bromide (a short acting acetylcholine esterase inhibitor) is injected intravenously after a 2 mg test dose. A positive result is indicated by an almost immediate, though short lived improvement in the weakness, ptosis and other signs. Serum may be tested for antibodies directed against the acetylcholine receptor on the muscle endplate. This is positive in at least 80% of cases. It is less likely to be positive in purely ocular cases, who may also have a negative Tensilon test. A chest X-ray or preferably a CT scan of the chest will help to exclude a thymoma, present in 10% of patients with myasthenia (usually middle aged men with the disease), and identify those with thymic hyperplasia. The vital capacity should be checked regularly morning and evening both lying and standing.

3. Initial therapy is with oral acetylcholine esterase inhibitors, pyridostigmine and neostigmine. Failing this thymectomy and/or steroids are used. If the problem is severe and other therapy unavailing, plasmapheresis combined with immune suppression is advocated.

7. A man of 52 years of age is admitted with a history of a major seizure at home. He is dysphasic but his wife gave a history that he had not been well for about five days with a high temperature and had been 'confused' for a day before his admission, which was precipitated by a major tonic clonic seizure. There is a past history of a major abdominal operation a few years previously from which he made a good recovery, he had been treated for mild hypertension over the last five years.

On examination, the man was pyrexial (38°C), restless and disorientated with a fluent dysphasia, possibly a right homonymous hemianopia and bilateral extensor plantar responses.

Investigations showed:

Blood
  Hb   13.8 g/dl
  WBC   11 x 10^9/l
  ESR   60 mm in first hour

Questions:

1. Give two possible diagnoses.

2. What investigations are needed to make the diagnosis?

3. What treatment is available for this condition?

Answers overleaf

Case Histories : Answers

7. 1. The combination of a major seizure with a pyrexia, confusion and focal neurological signs make the diagnosis of herpes simplex encephalitis (HSE) likely. An alternative would include a bacterial cerebral abscess, although this is less common.

2. The first essential investigation is an X-ray CT scan of the head to exclude a cerebral abscess or cerebritis. If encephalitis is the diagnosis, areas of low attenuation due to brain swelling or high attenuation areas of haemorrhagic necrosis may be present. However, the CT scan may be normal in HSE. The most sensitive test for the diagnosis of HSE is the EEG. This characteristically shows repetitive high voltage sharp and slow wave complexes in the temporal lobes, often bilateral and asymetrical. Once the CT scan has excluded a mass lesion, lumbar puncture should be performed, there being a moderate lymphocyte pleocytosis in HSE.

3. If HSE is suspected, acyclovir should be used intravenously for a minimum of ten days, the evidence suggesting that early use of this drug significantly improves the chances of functional recovery. Once a patient becomes comatose with HSE the outcome for full recovery is poor although with acyclovir the outcome is no longer hopeless. HSE is particularly likely to occur in patients with some degree of immune deficiency such as haematological malignancy.

NEUROLOGY : DATA INTERPRETATIONS

1. A 15 year old boy presented with a pyrexia, headache and neck stiffness but no focal neurological signs.
   The following is the blood picture and CSF analysis:
   CSF
       Pressure   190 mm H_2O
       Protein   0.36 g/l
       Cells   36/mm^3 lymphocytes
       Glucose   4 mmol/l
       Gram stain   no organisms seen
   Blood
       Hb   14.4 g/dl
       WBC   4 x 10^9/l, lymphocytes 45%
       ESR   30 mm in first hour
       Glucose   5.3 mmol/l

   Questions:
   1. What is the likely diagnosis?
   2. Name three organisms that commonly cause this problem.
   3. What less common disorders can produce this CSF picture.

2. A 28 year old publican presented with a pyrexia, neck stiffness, photophobia and mild optic disc swelling. He had had a splenectomy following a road traffic accident five years previously.
   The following is the blood picture and CSF analysis:

   CSF
       Pressure   280 mm H_2O
       Protein   1.2 g/l
       Cells   230 cells/mm^3, 85% polymorphonuclears
       Glucose   1.8 mmol/l
       Gram stains   occasional Gram positive diplococci
   Blood
       Hb   13.6 g/dl
       WBC   17 x 10^9/l, lymphocytes 13%
       ESR   80 mm in first hour
       Glucose   6.2 mmol/l

   Questions:
   1. What is the diagnosis?
   2. What initial treatment should be instituted?
   3. What is the prognosis?

Answers overleaf

Data Interpretations : Answers

1. 1. Acute viral meningitis.

   2. The most common organisms to cause this include echovirus coxsackie, mumps and the EB virus (infectious mononucleosis).

   3. Less common causes include leptospirosis, Q fever, leukaemic meningitis (unlikely here with the near normal blood picture and Behcet's disease (usually with a history of recurrent oro genital ulceration). Tuberculous meningitis and other chronic bacterial infections are unlikely in view of the normal CSF sugar level (usually greater than 40% of the blood sugar).

2. 1. Bacterial meningitis. In view of the history of splenectomy the likeliest organism is pneumococcus and the possibility of alcohol abuse (he is a publican) increases the risk of this organism. At his age the other likely organism is the meningococcus.

   2. Both of these organisms are sensitive to penicillin and this should be started at a dose of 1.2–2.4 g per 24 hours intravenously.

   3. The prognosis in pneumococcal meningitis associated with splenectomy is variable and patients may be left with substantial neurological deficit if treatment is not started very promptly. The presence of cerebral oedema (disc swelling) and focal signs (not present here) are poor prognosticants.

Neurology : Data Interpretations

3. A patient who recently returned from a four week visit to Poland presented with a mild headache, a sixth nerve palsy and slight ataxia.

These are the blood and CSF results:

CSF
    Pressure   305 mm H_2O
    Protein   2.1 g/l
    Cells   60/mm^3, 90% lymphocytes
    Glucose   0.6 mmol/l

Blood
    Hb   12.4 g/dl
    WBC   10 x 10^9/l, lymphocytes 33%
    Glucose   5.1 mmol/l

Questions:

1. What is the likely diagnosis?
2. What treatment should be started?
3. Give three complications which may arise.

4. A man of 34 years of age presented with a week's history of limb weakness, diplopia and mild papilloedema.

The CSF results below were obtained:

CSF
    Pressure   310 mm H_2O
    Protein   2.6 g/l
    Cells   5 lymphocytes/mm^3
    Glucose   4.8 mmol/l (blood glucose 5.4 mmol/l)

Questions:

1. What is the diagnosis?
2. What two further investigations would assist management?
3. Explain the mechanism involved in the presence of papilloedema?

Answers overleaf

Data Interpretations : Answers

3. 1. Lymphocytic meningitis with a low CSF sugar, raised protein and raised intracranial pressure. The likely cause is tuberculous meningitis, complicated by hydrocephalus. The ataxia is a sign of hydrocephalus, the sixth nerve palsy is either a false localising sign of the raised intracranial pressure or related to the basal meningitis. Sarcoid can cause a lymphocytic basal meningitis, but the CSF sugar is not usually so low.

2. In view of the CSF results and in advance of bacteriological confirmation anti-tuberculosis therapy should be started, probably with four drugs, rifampicin, isoniazid, pyrazinamide and ethambutol. If hydrocephalus is present and the conscious level declines, concomitant steroid therapy is recommended.

3. Complications other than hydrocephalus (identified by CT scanning) include spinal block, stroke due to endarteritis and the formation of tuberculomata.

4. 1. Guillain-Barré syndrome, showing typical normal cell count with very raised protein level and normal CSF glucose in a man with a progressive neuropathy, including cranial neuropathy.

2. Further investigation should include spirometry to measure lung vital capacity to identify neurogenic hypoventilation (blood gases deteriorate late in Guillain-Barré syndrome).

3. A syndrome resembling benign intracranial hypertension (pseudotumour cerebri) can occur in Guillain-Barré syndrome. The mechanism is thought to be blockage of the CSF absorption at the arachnoid villi by the very raised CSF protein.

Neurology : Data Interpretations

5. A woman of 35 years of age presented with a history of a mild paraparesis of three weeks duration. On her left alar nasae there was a 1 cm raised slightly purplish erythematous lesion of the skin.

At lumbar puncture the following results were obtained:

CSF
    Pressure   160 mm H_2O
    Protein   0.75 g/l
    Cells   85 lymphocytes/mm^3
    Glucose   3.8 mmol/l (blood glucose 4.2 mmol/l)

Questions:

1. What three investigations would further aid diagnosis?

2. What is the treatment?

3. What complications may arise?

6. A man of 25 years of age presents with a history of leg weakness and backache. He has birthmarks and poor vision of long standing in his left eye.

At myelogram investigations showed:

CSF
    Cells   3 lymphocytes/mm^3
    Protein   4.5 g/l
    Glucose   3.9 mmol/l (blood glucose 4.7 mmol/l)

Questions:

1. What did the myelogram show?

2. What other lesions may be present?

3. What is the cause of his visual difficulty?

Answers overleaf

Data Interpretations : Answers

5. 1. The likely diagnosis is sarcoidosis, the skin lesion described suggests lupus pernio. A useful investigation would be biopsy of the skin lesion. The lymphocyte count is rather high for myelitis from multiple sclerosis although this would be in the differential diagnosis. Visual evoked responses would aid diagnosis as would an MRI (magnetic resonance) scan of the head. Ophthalmological investigation may reveal sarcoid uveitis.

2. If sarcoidosis is confirmed treatment with steroids for six months is indicated, treatment progress being monitored by the disappearance of the lupus pernio.

3. Complications of intrathecal sarcoid include hydrocephalus from basal meningeal inflammation which may also provoke cranial nerve paresis, especially facial nerve lesions. Spinal radiculopathy may also occur.

6. 1. This is the CSF picture of spinal block. The skin lesions are probably 'cafe-au-lait' patches of neurofibromatosis. The myelogram showed complete extradural obstruction to contrast flow due to a thoracic neurofibroma.

2. Eighth nerve neurofibromata, intracerebral glioma and meningioma may be present as well as multiple spinal neurofibroma.

3. The visual loss is due to an optic nerve glioma, an indolent neoplasm, common in neurofibromatosis.

Neurology : Data Interpretations

7. A young woman who had presented with a history of intermittent blurred vision and who was found to have bilateral papilloedema. An unenhanced CT scan was normal.

Spinal fluid obtained showed:

CSF
- Pressure   450 mm H_2O
- Cells   2 lymphocytes/mm^3
- Protein   0.33 g/l
- Glucose   3.7 mmol/l (blood glucose 4/1 mmol/l)

Questions:

1. What is the diagnosis?

2. What three therapies are available?

3. What complications can occur?

8. A young forestry worker from Suffolk who had had a persistent recurrent rash on his leg for some weeks was admitted with multiple limb pains and bilateral facial weakness. His CT scan was normal. The following CSF results were obtained.

CSF
- Pressure   190 mm H_2O
- Cells   74/mm^3, 90% lymphocytes
- Protein   1.1 g/l
- Glucose   2.8 mmol/l (blood glucose 5.3 mmol/l)

Questions:

1. What is the diagnosis?

2. What other clinical feature may occur?

3. What is the treatment?

Answers overleaf

Data Interpretations : Answers

7. 1. Benign intracranial hypertension (pseudotumour cerebri) is the most likely diagnosis, a less likely possibility being venous sinus thrombosis. Benign intracranial hypertension is probably caused by defective reabsorption of CSF from the arachnoid villi.

2. Benign intracranial hypertension is often self-limiting and the initial therapy is the repeated removal of CSF by lumbar puncture. If this fails there is a risk to vision so either thecoperitoneal shunting or optic nerve decompression are indicated.

3. Apart from visual failure sixth nerve palsies may occur and act as false localising signs.

8. 1. Lyme disease, an infection by the spirochaete, *Borrelia burgdorferi* is the most likely diagnosis. The first clue is his occupation since this infection is found in ticks common in downland and wooded areas. The diagnostic combination is a lymphocytic meningitis with cranial polyneuropathy and a characteristic migratory erythematous rash. Confirmation of the disease can be made by detection of raised titres of a specific IgM antibody rising to a peak after six weeks. Sarcoidosis is in the differential diagnosis as are other causes of lymphocytic meningitis.

2. In addition to a meningitis with cranial and spinal radiculopathy there may be an arthritis.

3. The organism is sensitive to penicillin and tetracycline.

Neurology : Data Interpretations

9. A 43 year old television producer was admitted with a pyrexia, ataxia, dysarthria and slight drowsiness.

A CT scan was normal but the CSF showed the following changes:

CSF
- Pressure   210 mm H_2O
- Cells   83/mm^3, 80% polymorphonuclear cells
- Protein   0.75 g/l
- Glucose   2.1 mmol/l (blood glucose 4.2 mmol/l)

Questions:

1. What is the diagnosis?
2. What other investigation might be helpful?
3. What is the correct therapy?

10. A 53 year old woman presents with a history of numbness of the feet and gait difficulty. On examination tendon reflexes are absent, plantar responses bilaterally extensor and proprioception impaired in the lower limbs.

The following investigation results are obtained:
Blood
- Hb   11.6 g/dl
- MCV   103 fl
- WBC   8 x 10^9/l
- ESR   30 mm in first hour

Nerve conduction studies
- Sural sensory action potential (amplitude)   3 microvolts (N=>15)
- Radial nerve sensory action potential (amplitude)   5 microvolts (N=>20)
- Common peroneal nerve motor conduction velocity   48 m/sec (N=>45)

Questions:

1. What is the differential diagnosis? Give two.
2. What two further investigations are necessary?
3. What treatment is indicated?

Answers overleaf

81

Data Interpretations : Answers

9. 1. The most likely diagnosis is meningitis with rhombencephalitis (the brain stem signs), characteristic of listeriosis, and infection caused by *Listeria monocytogenes*. This most often causes infection in immunosuppressed patients and during pregnancy but not always.

2. Further investigation might include blood cultures since the organism is often easier to culture from blood than CSF.

3. Listeria is sensitive to ampicillin and this is usually indicated in high doses.

10. 1. The investigations show a combination of signs of peripheral neuropathy with some upper motor neurone signs and a macrocytosis. The nerve conduction tests show a reduction in sensory actional potential amplitude with normal motor conduction velocity, characteristic of an axonal neuropathy. The most likely diagnosis is pernicious anaemia with subacute combined degeneration of the cord and peripheral neuropathy. A history of alcoholism may indicate that the neuropathy is due to ethanol, though the extensor plantars would still need accounting for.

2. A Schilling test for vitamin B_{12} malabsorption is necessary. Antibodies to intrinsic factor may be present.

3. If vitamin B_{12} deficiency is present then replacement therapy is urgently required to prevent permanent disability.

Neurology : Data Interpretations

1. A 22 year old woman presents with bilateral foot drop, slowly worsening over the last five years. There is symmetrical distal wasting of all extremities, more pronounced in the lower limbs.

   The following neurophysiological results are obtained:

Radial nerve sensory action potential	<1 microvolt (N=>20)
Sural nerve sensory action potential	unobtainable (N=>15)
Median nerve motor conduction velocity	23 m/sec (N=>50)
Common peroneal nerve conduction velocity	15 m/sec (N=>45)

   ### Questions:

   1. What is the diagnosis?
   2. What would you advise this girl about having a family?
   3. What measure might help her disability?

2. A woman of 24 years of age has some difficulty seeing clearly out of one eye, describing her vision as misty.

   Visual evoked responses are obtained:

Left P100	98 msecs	(amplitude 12 microvolts) (upper limit of normal 107 msecs)
Right P100	120 msecs	(amplitude 5 microvolts)

   ### Questions:

   1. What is the cause of the visual problem?
   2. What is the prognosis for vision?
   3. Will other deficits complicate the picture?

Answers overleaf

Data Interpretations : Answers

11. 1. The history of prolonged progression since teenage years points to a congenital disorder. The nerve conduction tests show a marked degree of motor slowing suggesting a demyelinating neuropathy. She has the clinical picture of Charcot-Marie-Tooth disease and this, with the nerve conduction test results, suggests hereditary sensorimotor neuropathy (HSMN) type I. The same syndrome (though usually of later onset) may be caused by an axonal neuropathy (HSMN type II) in which case the motor conduction velocity is only mildly reduced; or by a spinal muscular atrophy in which case distal conduction is normal and sensory action potentials are present.

2. HSMN I is dominantly inherited and so if this is the diagnosis (neurophysiological tests of the parents and siblings may help), the patient must be advised that there is a 50% chance of her offspring developing the disorder although the phenotypic expression is variable.

3. Lightweight footdrop supports will improve her mobility.

12. 1. Optic neuritis. The P100 wave of the visual evoked response is usually around 100 msecs. Delay on the symptomatic side suggests optic nerve slowing due to demyelination.

2. Visual recovery is likely though the P100 may remain delayed.

3. 40–60% of patients who have an attack of optic neuritis go on to develop other features of multiple sclerosis, the risk being greater for those of tissue type HLA-DR2, those with more than one attack and winter onset of optic neuritis.

Neurology : Data Interpretations

13. A 10 year old boy is referred for investigation of educational and behavioural difficulties of recent onset. He is found to be unsteady on his feet and has a few involuntary jerking movements of his limbs.

    Investigations provided the following:

Head CT:	Normal
EEG:	Periodic (4 Hz) high voltage sharp and slow complexes
CSF:	No cells
Protein	0.86 g/l (raised gamma-globulin)

    Questions:

    1. What is the diagnosis?
    2. What is the aetiology of this disorder?
    3. What outcome is likely?

14. A chronically depressed 38 year old woman with a past history of alcohol abuse has been in hospital a few days for investigation of abdominal pain when she becomes ataxic and confused. On examination reflexes are difficult to obtain and nystagmus is present.

    The following investigations are obtained:

Head CT scan	Normal
CSF	Normal

    Blood
Hb	13.7 g/dl
MCV	101 fl
WBC	11 x 10^9/l
ESR	38 mm in first hour

    Questions:

    1. What is the diagnosis?
    2. What other investigation may confirm this diagnosis?
    3. What treatment is indicated?

Answers overleaf

Data Interpretations : Answers

13. 1. Subacute sclerosing panencephalitis (SSPE) is the most likely diagnosis. This is a rare late complication of measles infection (or even less frequently measles vaccination). There is a relentlessly progressive dementia with ataxia and myoclonus. The EEG appearances are characteristic.

2. There is an oligoclonal electrophoretic pattern of gamma-globulin which cross reacts with the measles virus antigen. The pathogenesis is thought to be a hyperimmune reaction to persistent measles antigen.

3. The outcome is uniformly poor, death in inanition coming after several years of progressive deficit.

14. 1. The raised MCV confirms this woman is still drinking, so Wernicke's encephalopathy in a chronic alcoholic is the most likely diagnosis. The combination of thiamine deficiency with carbohydrate intake (following hospitalisation) produces haemorrhagic necrosis in the limbic system especially the mammillary bodies and rostral brainstem. The triad of ataxia, confusion and nystagmus is diagnostic.

2. Estimation of the red cell transketolase may allow biochemical confirmation of the diagnosis.

3. Treatment with intravenous thiamine will resolve the syndrome in most cases if applied in time, although there may be residual cognitive impairment.

INDEX

acyclovir 72
adhesive capsulitis 56
AIDS 32
alcoholism 18, 82
anaemia
    iron deficiency 22
    macrocytic 18, 24
    microcytic hypochromic 12
arthritis
    acute sarcoid 44
    pyrophosphate 30
    rheumatoid 34

cancer
    breast 66
    lung 4
Charcot-Marie-Tooth disease 84

dermatomyositis 52
disseminated intravascular coagulation 20

encephalitis, herpes simplex 72
epilepsy 62

folate deficiency 24, 28

glomerulonephritis, acute 42
gout 38

haemochromatosis 30
    idiopathic 8
haemolysis, immune mediated 24
heparin 26
hereditary sensorimotor neuropathy 84
Hodgkin's disease 2
hypertension 6
    benign intracranial 80

iron deficiency 12

leukaemia
    acute 4, 14
listeriosis 82

liver disease, alcoholic 8
lupus pernio 78
Lyme disease 36, 80
lymphoma, non-Hodgkin's 2

measles 86
α-methyldopa 24
meningioma 66
meningitis 82
    bacterial 74
    lymphocytic 76
    viral 74
multiple myelomatosis 12, 54
multiple sclerosis 66, 84
myasthenia gravis 34, 64, 70

neurofibroma 66
neurofibromatosis 78

optic neuritis 84

Paget's disease 50
parvovirus 16
pernicious anaemia 82
pneumonia 4, 34
polycythaemia rubra vera 28

sarcoidosis 78
septrin 28
sickle cell disease 18
spherocytosis, hereditary 16
Still's disease 48
subacute sclerosing panencephalitis 86
subdural haematoma 60
syndrome
    antiphospholipid 36
    Brown-Sequard 68
    carpal tunnel 70
    Guillain-Barré 64, 76
    hypermobility 58
    Löfgren's 44
    lupus 40
    Sjögren's 46

Index

systemic lupus erythematosus 36, 42

thalassaemia 18, 22
thrombocythaemia, essential 10
transfusion reaction 22

tuberculosis 2

vitamin B12 deficiency 18

Wegener's granulomatosis 30
Wernicke's encephalopathy 86
Whipple's disease 32